Ninja Speedi Cookb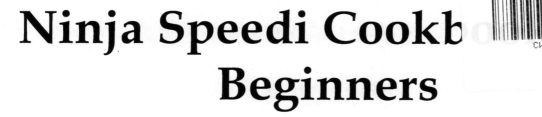 Beginners

Unlock the Secrets of Ultra-Fast Cooking with the Ninja Speedi CookBook!. Easy, Healthy and Delicious Recipes For Beginners To Air Fry, Bake, Roast Everyday.

Charlotte Morley

Table of Contents

Introduction

Welcome to the Ninja Speedi CookBook! This cookbook is designed to help you get the most out of your Ninja kitchen appliances, and to make your mealtimes easier, healthier and more enjoyable. If you're a beginner, this cookbook features a wide range of recipes that will help you make the most of your Ninja kitchen appliances. You'll find delicious meals that can be prepared quickly and easily, making use of the unique features of the Ninja kitchen appliances, such as the custom programs, pre-set temperatures, and manual settings. Inside this cookbook, you'll find recipes for everything from breakfast, main dishes to desserts, snacks, and Sides. We've included recipes for both traditional and modern dishes, so no matter what your tastes, you're sure to find something to satisfy your hunger.

The Ninja Speedi Rapid Cooker is a revolutionary kitchen appliance that is designed to make cooking easier. With its unique and innovative features, the Ninja Speedi Rapid Cooker will help you save time and energy while creating delicious meals. Before you begin cooking with your Ninja Speedi Rapid Cooker, there are a few steps you should take. First, familiarize yourself with the appliance by reading the user manual. This will provide you with detailed instructions and safety tips for using the Ninja Speedi Rapid Cooker. Next, choose the correct size pot for your food. The Ninja Speedi Rapid Cooker comes in two sizes - 4.5 liters and 6 liters, and the size of pot you need will depend on the amount of food you're cooking. Once you've selected the correct pot size, it's time to begin cooking. The Ninja Speedi Rapid Cooker comes with three heat settings - low, medium, and high. Before you select your heat setting, decide what type of food you are cooking and adjust the heat accordingly. For example, if you're cooking a stew you would want to use the low setting, while a stir fry may require the high setting. Next, select the appropriate cooking time. The Ninja Speedi Rapid Cooker has two main settings - slow cook and quick cook. Slow cook is ideal for slow-cooked dishes such as soups, stews, and braised meats, while quick cook is perfect for quick-cooking items such as vegetables and rice.

The recipes in this cookbook are designed to be nutritious and delicious, and they're perfect for busy people who don't have time to spend hours in the kitchen. We've included tips and tricks to help you make the most of your time, and to help you produce meals that are both healthy and delicious.

Ninja Speedi Cooking Basics and Tips

1. Pre-heat the pan: Pre-heating the pan before you start to cook is essential for Ninja Speedi Cooking. It helps to evenly circulate the heat and prevents food from sticking to the pan.

2. Use cooking oils: Choose a good quality cooking oil that can withstand high heat. This will help your food cook faster and also provide flavor.

3. Cook food in batches: Cooking food in batches is a great way to speed up the cooking process. This will also ensure that all the food is cooked evenly and quickly.

4. Use high heat: High heat is essential for Ninja Speedi Cooking. This will help to cook the food quickly and evenly.

5. Use a timer: A timer is essential for Ninja Speedi Cooking. It will help you to keep track of the cooking time and ensure that the food is cooked properly.

6. Use fresh ingredients: Fresh ingredients are essential for Ninja Speedi Cooking. They are more flavorful and cook quicker than frozen or canned ingredients.

7. Use a pressure cooker: Pressure cookers are a great tool for Ninja Speedi Cooking. They help to cook food quickly and evenly, and can be used for a variety of dishes.

8. Use a food processor: A food processor is a great tool for Ninja Speedi Cooking. It can help to quickly and easily chop, dice, and mince ingredients, as well as mix batters and sauces.

9. Plan ahead: Planning ahead is essential for Ninja Speedi Cooking. Ensure you have all the ingredients you need and that you have a good idea of the steps you need to take to make a dish.

10. Clean as you go: Cleaning as you go is essential for Ninja Speedi Cooking. This will help to keep the kitchen clean and organized and make the cooking process much easier.

Follow these tips and you will be able to whip up delicious meals in no time!

Benefits of Ninja Speedi Rapid Cooker

1. Quick Cooking Times: The Ninja Speedi Rapid Cooker cooks food up to 70% faster than traditional cooking methods, allowing you to enjoy a meal in a fraction of the time.

2. Versatile: The Ninja Speedi Rapid Cooker can be used to steam, bake, sauté, and slow cook a variety of dishes. It can even roast a whole chicken in under an hour.

3. Easy to Use: With its intuitive digital display, the Ninja Speedi Rapid Cooker is easy to use and requires minimal preparation time.

4. Healthy: The Ninja Speedi Rapid Cooker locks in vitamins and minerals, preserving the flavor and nutrition of your favorite dishes.

5. Convenient: The Ninja Speedi Rapid Cooker is a space-saving kitchen appliance that can be used to cook entire meals. It also features a delay start timer, so you can set it up before you leave for work and have a hot meal waiting for you when you get home.

How to Use the Ninja Speedi Rapid Cooker

The Ninja Speedi Rapid Cooker lets you simultaneously cook two different meals using the same cooking function, and you can do so by using the elevated and bottom positions inside the cooking pot. The crisper tray that goes inside the cooker can be set in an elevated position to add food to a second layer. For conventional steam and air frying, use the bottom position. To position the Crisper Tray in the raised position, turn the tray's legs outward until they protrude past each of the tray's four corners. The tray should stay upright in the pot by resting on the legs, which should rest on the ledges at the bottom of each groove.

Carefully add any necessary ingredients to the bottom of the pot before elevating the Crisper Tray. The Crisper Tray must be placed in an elevated position when using recipes that call for the Speedi Meals feature. Rotate the Crisper Tray's legs inward so that they are pressed up against the tray's underside to position it in the bottom position. As a result, the Crisper Tray will be able to rest at the base of the pot.

Cleaning & Maintenance

After each session of cooking, the appliance needs to be completely cleaned. Before washing, unplug the appliance from the wall socket and make sure it is completely cool. Wipe a moist towel over the control panel and cooker base to clean them. The dishwasher can be used to clean the entire dinner pot, crisper tray, and condensation catch. Fill the pot with water and let soak before cleaning if food residue is stuck to the pot or crisper tray. Avoid using scouring pads. If scrubbing is required, use a nylon pad or brush with liquid dish soap or non-abrasive cleaner.

Cleaning the Lid

Prior to using the "wet cooking functions," which include the Slow Cook, Sous Vide, Sear/Sauté, and all Rapid Cooker settings, I would recommend you check the interior of the lid. I advise cleaning the appliance, followed by wiping down the interior of the lid to prevent burning if you notice any food residue or oil buildup on the heating element or fan.

Steam Cleaning

Add three cups of water to the pot. Change the Smart Switch to the Rapid Cooker. Set the timer to 10 minutes and choose STEAM. Use any damp cloth or sponge to clean the interior of the lid once the clock hits zero and the device has cooled. Avoid touching the fan when cleaning the lid's interior. To make sure all residue has been removed, drain the water from the pot and rinse both the cooking pot and the crisper tray.

CHAPTER 1: Breakfast Recipes

1. Sausage and Egg Casserole

Preparation Time: 10 minutes

Cooking Time: 20 minutes

Servings: 4

Ingredients:

- 12 oz. breakfast sausage
- 6 eggs
- 1/2 cup shredded cheese
- 1/2 cup milk
- 1/2 cup chopped onions
- 1/2 cup diced bell peppers
- 1/2 cup diced mushrooms
- Salt and pepper to taste

Directions:

1. Place the sausage in the Ninja Speedi Rapid Cooker.
2. Add eggs, cheese, milk, onions, bell peppers, mushrooms, and salt and pepper.
3. Close the lid and set the timer for 10 minutes.
4. When the timer goes off, open the lid and give the casserole a gentle stir.
5. Close the lid and set the timer for an additional 10 minutes.
6. When the timer goes off, open the lid and serve.

Nutrition: Calories: 299kcal; Fat: 8.8g; Carb: 10g; Protein: 11.64g

2. Bacon and Cheese Omelet

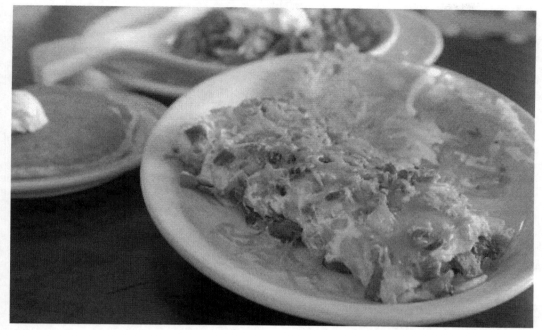

Preparation Time: 10 minutes

Cooking Time: 15 minutes

Servings: 4

Ingredients:

- 4 slices of bacon, diced
- 4 eggs
- 1/2 cup shredded cheese
- 2 tablespoons milk
- Salt and pepper to taste

Directions:

1. Place the bacon in the Ninja Speedi Rapid Cooker.
2. Add the eggs, cheese, milk, salt and pepper.
3. Close the lid and set the timer for 10 minutes.
4. When the timer goes off, open the lid and gently stir the omelet.
5. Close the lid and set the timer for an additional 5 minutes.
6. When the timer goes off, open the lid and serve.

Nutrition: Calories: 206kcal; Fat: 8.8g; Carb: 12g; Protein: 9.64g

3. French Toast

Preparation Time: 10 minutes

Cooking Time: 15 minutes

Servings: 4

Ingredients:

- 4 slices of bread
- 2 eggs
- 1/2 cup milk
- 2 tablespoons sugar
- 1 teaspoon vanilla extract
- 1/2 teaspoon cinnamon
- Pinch of salt

Directions:

1. Place the bread in the Ninja Speedi Rapid Cooker.
2. In another bowl, whisk together the eggs, milk, sugar, vanilla extract, cinnamon, and salt.
3. Pour the egg mixture over the bread.
4. Close the lid and set the timer for 10 minutes.
5. When the timer goes off, open the lid and gently stir the French toast.
6. Close the lid and set the timer for an additional 5 minutes.
7. When the timer goes off, open the lid and serve.

Nutrition: Calories: 300kcal; Fat: 10.8g; Carb: 15g; Protein: 11.64g

4. Pancakes

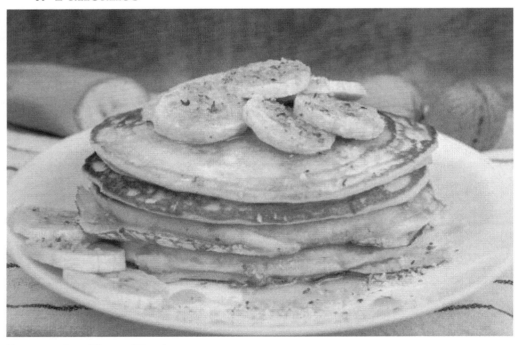

Preparation Time: 10 minutes

Cooking Time: 15 minutes

Servings: 4

Ingredients:

- 1 cup all-purpose flour
- 2 teaspoons baking powder
- 1/2 teaspoon salt
- 1 tablespoon sugar
- 1 cup milk
- 2 tablespoons butter, melted
- 1 egg

Directions:

1. Place the flour, baking powder, salt, and sugar in the Ninja Speedi Rapid Cooker.
2. Add the milk, butter, and egg and mix until well combined.
3. Close the lid and set the timer for 10 minutes.
4. When the timer goes off, open the lid and gently stir the pancake batter.
5. Close the lid and set the timer for an additional 5 minutes.
6. When the timer goes off, open the lid and serve.

Nutrition: Calories: 299kcal; Fat: 9.8g; Carb: 19g; Protein: 12.64g

5. Egg and Vegetable Frittata

Preparation Time: 10 minutes

Cooking Time: 20 minutes

Servings: 4

Ingredients:

- 8 eggs
- 1/2 cup shredded cheese
- 1/2 cup diced onions
- 1/2 cup diced bell peppers
- 1/2 cup diced mushrooms
- 1/4 cup milk
- Salt and pepper to taste

Directions:

1. Place the eggs, cheese, onions, bell peppers, mushrooms, milk, and salt and pepper in the Ninja Speedi Rapid Cooker.
2. Close the lid and set the timer for 10 minutes.
3. When the timer goes off, open the lid and gently stir the frittata.
4. Close the lid and set the timer for an additional 10 minutes.
5. When the timer goes off, open the lid and serve.

Nutrition: Calories: 211kcal; Fat: 8.8g; Carb: 14g; Protein: 12.64g

6. Breakfast Burrito

Preparation Time: 10 minutes

Cooking Time: 15 minutes

Servings: 4

Ingredients:

- 1 cup cooked sausage
- 4 eggs
- 1/2 cup cooked rice
- 1/2 cup shredded cheese
- 1/2 cup diced tomatoes
- 1/2 cup diced onion
- 1/2 cup diced bell peppers
- 1/4 cup salsa
- Salt and pepper to taste

Directions:

1. Place the sausage, eggs, rice, cheese, tomatoes, onion, bell peppers, salsa, and salt and pepper in the Ninja Speedi Rapid Cooker.
2. Close the lid and set the timer for 10 minutes.
3. When the timer goes off, open the lid and gently stir the burrito filling.
4. Close the lid and set the timer for an additional 5 minutes.
5. When the timer goes off, open the lid and serve.

Nutrition: Calories: 321kcal; Fat: 8.8g; Carb: 20g; Protein: 11.64g

7. Hash Brown Casserole

Preparation Time: 5 minutes

Cooking Time: 20 minutes

Servings: 4

Ingredients:

- 2 cups shredded hash brown potatoes
- 1/2 cup shredded cheese
- 1/2 cup diced onions
- 1/2 cup diced bell peppers
- 4 eggs
- 1/4 cup milk
- Salt and pepper to taste

Directions:

1. Place the hash browns, cheese, onions, bell peppers, eggs, milk, and salt and pepper in the Ninja Speedi Rapid Cooker.
2. Close the lid and set the timer for 10 minutes.
3. When the timer goes off, open the lid and give the casserole a gentle stir.
4. Close the lid and set the timer for an additional 10 minutes.
5. When the timer goes off, open the lid and serve.

Nutrition: Calories: 287kcal; Fat: 8.8g; Carb: 15g; Protein: 13.64g

8. Bacon and Egg Quiche

Preparation Time: 10 minutes

Cooking Time: 20 minutes

Servings: 4

Ingredients:

- 4 slices of bacon, diced
- 4 eggs
- 1 cup shredded cheese
- 1/2 cup milk
- 1/2 cup diced onions
- 1/2 cup diced bell peppers
- Salt and pepper to taste

Directions:

1. Place the bacon in the Ninja Speedi Rapid Cooker.
2. Add the eggs, cheese, milk, onions, bell peppers, and salt and pepper.
3. Close the lid and set the timer for 10 minutes.
4. When the timer goes off, open the lid and gently stir the quiche.
5. Close the lid and set the timer for an additional 10 minutes.
6. When the timer goes off, open the lid and serve.

Nutrition: Calories: 300kcal; Fat: 8.8g; Carb: 10g; Protein: 11.64g

9. Breakfast Burrito Bowl

Preparation Time: 10 minutes

Cooking Time: 15 minutes

Servings: 4

Ingredients:

- 1 cup cooked sausage
- 4 eggs

- 1/2 cup cooked black beans
- 1/2 cup cooked rice
- 1/2 cup shredded cheese
- 1/2 cup diced tomatoes
- 1/2 cup diced onion
- 1/2 cup diced bell peppers
- 1/4 cup salsa
- Salt and pepper to taste

Directions:

1. Place the sausage, eggs, black beans, rice, cheese, tomatoes, onion, bell peppers, salsa, and salt and pepper in the Ninja Speedi Rapid Cooker.
2. Close the lid and set the timer for 10 minutes.
3. When the timer goes off, open the lid and gently stir the burrito bowl.
4. Close the lid and set the timer for an additional 5 minutes.
5. When the timer goes off, open the lid and serve.

Nutrition: Calories: 297kcal; Fat: 9.8g; Carb: 12g; Protein: 11.64g

10. Egg and Bacon Sandwich

Preparation Time: 5 minutes

Cooking Time: 15 minutes

Servings: 4

Ingredients:

- 4 slices of bacon, diced
- 4 eggs
- 2 slices of bread
- 1/4 cup shredded cheese
- Salt and pepper to taste

Directions:

1. Place the bacon in the Ninja Speedi Rapid Cooker.
2. Add the eggs, bread, cheese, and salt and pepper.
3. Close the lid and set the timer for 10 minutes.
4. When the timer goes off, open the lid and gently stir the sandwich filling.
5. Close the lid and set the timer for an additional 5 minutes.
6. When the timer goes off, open the lid and serve.

Nutrition: Calories: 265kcal; Fat: 8.8g; Carb: 10g; Protein: 11.64g

11. Breakfast Pizza

Preparation Time: 10 minutes

Cooking Time: 20 minutes

Servings: 4

Ingredients:

- 4 eggs
- 1/2 cup shredded cheese
- 1/2 cup diced onions
- 1/2 cup diced bell peppers
- 1/2 cup diced mushrooms
- 1 cup pizza sauce
- 1/2 cup shredded mozzarella cheese
- Salt and pepper to taste

Directions:

1. Place the eggs, cheese, onions, bell peppers, mushrooms, pizza sauce, and salt and pepper in the Ninja Speedi Rapid Cooker.
2. Close the lid and set the timer for 10 minutes.
3. When the timer goes off, open the lid and gently stir the pizza filling.
4. Top with the mozzarella cheese and close the lid.
5. Set the timer for an additional 5 minutes.
6. When the timer goes off, open the lid and serve.

Nutrition: Calories: 265kcal; Fat: 8.8g; Carb: 18g; Protein: 15.64g

12. Breakfast Tacos

Preparation Time: 10 minutes

Cooking Time: 15 minutes

Servings: 4

Ingredients:

- 1 cup cooked sausage
- 4 eggs
- 4 taco shells
- 1/2 cup shredded cheese
- 1/2 cup diced tomatoes
- 1/2 cup diced onion
- 1/2 cup diced bell peppers
- 1/4 cup salsa

- Salt and pepper to taste

Directions:

1. Place the sausage, eggs, cheese, tomatoes, onion, bell peppers, salsa, and salt and pepper in the Ninja Speedi Rapid Cooker.
2. Close the lid and set the timer for 10 minutes.
3. When the timer goes off, open the lid and gently stir the taco filling.
4. Close the lid and set the timer for an additional 5 minutes.
5. When the timer goes off, open the lid and serve over the taco shells.

Nutrition: Calories: 297kcal; Fat: 8.8g; Carb: 18g; Protein: 11.64g

13. Breakfast Sausage and Egg Sandwich

Preparation Time: 10 minutes

Cooking Time: 15 minutes

Servings: 4

Ingredients:

- 12 oz. breakfast sausage
- 4 eggs
- 2 slices of bread
- 1/2 cup shredded cheese
- Salt and pepper to taste

Directions:

1. Place the sausage in the Ninja Speedi Rapid Cooker.
2. Add the eggs, bread, cheese, and salt and pepper.
3. Close the lid and set the timer for 10 minutes.
4. When the timer goes off, open the lid and gently stir the sandwich filling.
5. Close the lid and set the timer for an additional 5 minutes.
6. When the timer goes off, open the lid and serve.

Nutrition: Calories: 221kcal; Fat: 8.8g; Carb: 10g; Protein: 9.64g

14. Biscuits and Gravy

Preparation Time: 10 minutes

Cooking Time: 15 minutes

Servings: 4

Ingredients:

- 1/2 cup all-purpose flour
- 2 tablespoons butter
- 2 cups milk

- 1/2 teaspoon salt
- 1/4 teaspoon pepper
- 1/4 teaspoon garlic powder
- 1/4 teaspoon onion powder
- 4 cooked biscuits

Directions:

1. Place the flour and butter in the Ninja Speedi Rapid Cooker.
2. Add the milk, salt, pepper, garlic powder, and onion powder and mix until well combined.
3. Close the lid and set the timer for 10 minutes.
4. When the timer goes off, open the lid and give the gravy a gentle stir.
5. Close the lid and set the timer for an additional 5 minutes.
6. When the timer goes off, open the lid and serve over the cooked biscuits.

Nutrition: Calories: 311kcal; Fat: 8.8g; Carb: 17g; Protein: 11.64g

15. Breakfast Quesadilla

Preparation Time: 10 minutes

Cooking Time: 15 minutes

Servings: 4

Ingredients:

- 4 eggs
- 4 flour tortillas
- 1/2 cup shredded cheese
- 1/2 cup diced tomatoes
- 1/2 cup diced onions
- 1/2 cup diced bell peppers
- 1/4 cup salsa
- Salt and pepper to taste

Directions:

1. Place the eggs, cheese, tomatoes, onions, bell peppers, salsa, and salt and pepper in the Ninja Speedi Rapid Cooker.
2. Close the lid and set the timer for 10 minutes.
3. When the timer goes off, open the lid and gently stir the quesadilla filling.
4. Place a tortilla in the bottom of the Ninja Speedi Rapid Cooker and spread the filling over the tortilla.
5. Top with another tortilla and close the lid.
6. Set the timer for an additional 5 minutes.
7. When the timer goes off, open the lid and serve.

Nutrition: Calories: 299kcal; Fat: 8.8g; Carb: 10g; Protein: 11.64g

16. Overnight Oats

Preparation Time: 10 minutes

Cooking Time: 15 minutes

Servings: 4

Ingredients:

- 1/2 cup rolled oats
- 1/2 cup milk
- 2 tablespoons chia seeds
- 2 tablespoons honey
- 1/2 teaspoon cinnamon
- Pinch of salt

Directions:

1. Place the oats, milk, chia seeds, honey, cinnamon, and salt in the Ninja Speedi Rapid Cooker.
2. Close the lid and set the timer for 10 minutes.
3. When the timer goes off, open the lid and give the oats a gentle stir.
4. Close the lid and set the timer for an additional 5 minutes.
5. When the timer goes off, open the lid and serve.

Nutrition: Calories: 256kcal; Fat: 8.8g; Carb: 10g; Protein: 11.64g

17. Breakfast Parfait

Preparation Time: 10 minutes

Cooking Time: 10 minutes

Servings: 4

Ingredients:

- 1/2 cup rolled oats
- 1/2 cup Greek yogurt
- 2 tablespoons honey
- 1/2 teaspoon cinnamon
- 1/2 cup fresh fruit
- 2 tablespoons chopped nuts

Directions:

1. Place the oats, yogurt, honey, and cinnamon in the Ninja Speedi Rapid Cooker.
2. Close the lid and set the timer for 10 minutes.
3. When the timer goes off, open the lid and give the oats a gentle stir.
4. Place the fresh fruit and chopped nuts in the bottom of a bowl.
5. Top with the oat mixture and serve.

Nutrition: Calories: 278kcal; Fat: 6.8g; Carb: 16g; Protein: 11.64g

18. Breakfast Potatoes

Preparation Time: 10 minutes

Cooking Time: 20 minutes

Servings: 4

Ingredients:

- 2 cups diced potatoes
- 1/2 cup diced onions
- 1/2 cup diced bell peppers
- 2 tablespoons olive oil
- 1 teaspoon garlic powder
- 1 teaspoon onion powder
- Salt and pepper to taste

Directions:

1. Place the potatoes, onions, bell peppers, olive oil, garlic powder, onion powder, and salt and pepper in the Ninja Speedi Rapid Cooker.
2. Close the lid and set the timer for 10 minutes.
3. When the timer goes off, open the lid and give the potatoes a gentle stir.
4. Close the lid and set the timer for an additional 10 minutes.
5. When the timer goes off, open the lid and serve.

Nutrition: Calories: 299kcal; Fat: 5.8g; Carb: 10g; Protein: 11.64g

19. Breakfast Stuffed Peppers

Preparation Time: 10 minutes

Cooking Time: 20 minutes

Servings: 4

Ingredients:

- 4 bell peppers, tops removed
- 4 eggs
- 1/2 cup cooked sausage
- 1/2 cup cooked rice
- 1/2 cup shredded cheese
- 1/2 cup diced tomatoes
- 1/2 cup diced onion
- 1/2 cup diced bell peppers
- 1/4 cup salsa

- Salt and pepper to taste

Directions:

1. Place the eggs, sausage, rice, cheese, tomatoes, onion, bell peppers, salsa, and salt and pepper in the Ninja Speedi Rapid Cooker.
2. Close the lid and set the timer for 10 minutes.
3. When the timer goes off, open the lid and gently stir the stuffing.
4. Place the bell peppers in the Ninja Speedi Rapid Cooker and stuff with the filling.
5. Close the lid and set the timer for an additional 10 minutes.
6. When the timer goes off, open the lid and serve.

Nutrition: Calories: 299kcal; Fat: 8.8g; Carb: 16g; Protein: 9.64g

20. Breakfast Hash

Preparation Time: 5 minutes

Cooking Time: 20 minutes

Servings: 4

Ingredients:

- 2 cups diced potatoes
- 1/2 cup diced onions
- 1/2 cup diced bell peppers
- 1/2 cup cooked sausage
- 2 tablespoons olive oil
- 1 teaspoon garlic powder
- 1 teaspoon onion powder
- Salt and pepper to taste

Directions:

1. Place the potatoes, onions, bell peppers, sausage, olive oil, garlic powder, onion powder, and salt and pepper in the Ninja Speedi Rapid Cooker.
2. Close the lid and set the timer for 10 minutes.
3. When the timer goes off, open the lid and give the hash a gentle stir.
4. Close the lid and set the timer for an additional 10 minutes.
5. When the timer goes off, open the lid and serve.

Nutrition: Calories: 299kcal; Fat: 8.8g; Carb: 10g; Protein: 11.64g

CHAPTER 2: Appetizers and Snacks

21.Spinach Artichoke Dip

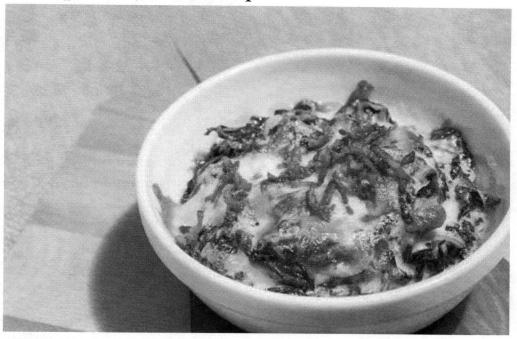

Preparation Time: 5 minutes

Cooking Time: 20 minutes

Servings: 4

Ingredients:

- 2 (14-ounce) cans artichoke hearts, drained and chopped
- 2 (10-ounce) packages frozen chopped spinach, thawed and drained
- 1 1/2 cups shredded mozzarella cheese
- 1 cup grated Parmesan cheese
- 1/2 cup sour cream
- 1/2 cup mayonnaise
- 2 cloves garlic, minced
- 1 teaspoon dried oregano
- 1/2 teaspoon red pepper flakes
- Salt and freshly ground black pepper

Directions:

1. Preheat the Ninja Speedi Rapid Cooker to 350 degrees F.
2. In a large bowl, combine the artichoke hearts, spinach, mozzarella cheese, Parmesan cheese, sour cream, mayonnaise, garlic, oregano, red pepper flakes, and salt and pepper to taste.

3. Transfer the dip to a greased 8-inch baking dish.

4. Conceal the dish with aluminum foil and bake in preheated Ninja Speedi Rapid Cooker for 20 minutes, or until hot and bubbly.

Nutrition: Calories: 546kcal; Fat: 20.8g; Carb: 22g; Protein: 18.64g

22.   Buffalo Chicken Dip

Preparation Time: 5 minutes

Cooking Time: 20 minutes

Servings: 4

Ingredients:

- 1 (12-ounce) package cream cheese, softened
- 1 (10-ounce) can chicken, drained
- 1/2 cup buffalo wing sauce
- 1/4 cup ranch dressing
- 1/4 cup crumbled blue cheese
- 1/4 cup shredded cheddar cheese
- 2 tablespoons chopped green onions

Directions:

1. Preheat the Ninja Speedi Rapid Cooker to 350 degrees F.

2. In a large basin, combine the cream cheese, chicken, buffalo wing sauce, ranch dressing, blue cheese, and cheddar cheese until well blended.

3. Spread the mixture into a greased 8-inch baking dish.

4. Conceal with aluminum foil and bake in the preheated Ninja Speedi Rapid Cooker for 20 minutes, or until hot and bubbly.

5. Sprinkle with the green onions before serving.

Nutrition: Calories: 467kcal; Fat: 34.1g; Carb: 11g; Protein: 28.64g

23.   Sweet and Spicy Sausage Bites

Preparation Time: 5 minutes

Cooking Time: 20 minutes

Servings: 4

Ingredients:

- 1 (16-ounce) package smoked sausage, cut into 1-inch pieces
- 1/2 cup dark brown sugar
- 1/4 cup honey

- 1/4 cup prepared yellow mustard
- 1/4 cup ketchup
- 1/4 teaspoon ground black pepper

Directions:

1. Preheat the Ninja Speedi Rapid Cooker to 350 degrees F.
2. Place the sausage pieces in a greased 8-inch baking dish.
3. In a medium bowl, whisk together the brown sugar, honey, mustard, ketchup, and pepper.
4. Pour the mixture over the sausage pieces and mix until evenly coated.
5. Conceal the dish with aluminum foil and bake in the preheated Ninja Speedi Rapid Cooker for 20 minutes, or until the sausage is cooked through.

Nutrition: Calories: 459kcal; Fat: 33.3g; Carb: 28g; Protein: 12.64g

24.   Bacon Wrapped Jalapeno Poppers

Preparation Time: 5 minutes

Cooking Time: 20 minutes

Servings: 4

Ingredients:

- 12 jalapeno peppers, halved and seeded
- 8 ounces cream cheese, softened
- 1/2 cup shredded cheddar cheese
- 1/4 cup chopped green onions
- 12 slices bacon, cut in half

Directions:

1. Preheat the Ninja Speedi Rapid Cooker to 350 degrees F.
2. In a medium basin, mix together the cream cheese, cheddar cheese, and green onions.
3. Spoon the mixture into the jalapeno pepper halves.
4. Wrap each jalapeno pepper half with a half slice of bacon and secure with a toothpick.
5. Place the bacon wrapped jalapeno poppers in a greased 8-inch baking dish.
6. Conceal the dish with aluminum foil and bake in the preheated Ninja Speedi Rapid Cooker for 20 minutes, or until the bacon is cooked through.

Nutrition: Calories: 519kcal; Fat: 41.8g; Carb: 12g; Protein: 23.64g

25.   Stuffed Mushrooms

Preparation Time: 5 minutes

Cooking Time: 20 minutes

Servings: 4

Ingredients:

- 20 large mushrooms, stems removed
- 2 tablespoons butter, melted
- 2 cloves garlic, minced
- 1/4 cup minced onion
- 1/4 cup grated Parmesan cheese
- 1/4 cup Italian-style bread crumbs
- 2 tablespoons chopped fresh parsley
- Salt and freshly ground black pepper

Directions:

1. Preheat the Ninja Speedi Rapid Cooker to 350 degrees F.
2. Place the mushrooms in a greased 8-inch baking dish.
3. In a medium bowl, mix together the butter, garlic, onion, Parmesan cheese, bread crumbs, parsley, and salt and pepper to taste.
4. Spoon the mixture into the mushroom caps.
5. Conceal the dish with aluminum foil and bake in the preheated Ninja Speedi Rapid Cooker for 20 minutes, or until the mushrooms are tender.

Nutrition: Calories: 150kcal; Fat: 8.8g; Carb: 11g; Protein: 6.9g

26.   Baked Potato Skins

Preparation Time: 15 minutes

Cooking Time: 1 hour 8 minutes

Servings: 4

Ingredients:

- 4 large baking potatoes
- 2 tablespoons olive oil
- 1/2 teaspoon garlic powder
- 1/2 teaspoon smoked paprika
- Salt and freshly ground black pepper
- 1/2 cup shredded cheddar cheese
- 1/4 cup sour cream
- 1/4 cup chopped green onions

Directions:

Preheat the Ninja Speedi Rapid Cooker to 350 degrees F.

Pierce the potatoes with a fork and rub with the olive oil. Sprinkle with the garlic powder, smoked paprika, and salt and pepper to taste.

Place potatoes on a baking sheet and bake in the preheated Ninja Speedi Rapid Cooker for 1 hour, or until tender.

Slice the potatoes in half and scoop out the insides, leaving a 1/4-inch thick shell.

Place the potato skins back on the baking sheet and top with the cheddar cheese.

Bake in the preheated Ninja Speedi Rapid Cooker for 8 minutes, or until the cheese is melted.

Top with the sour cream and green onions before serving.

Nutrition: Calories: 307kcal; Fat: 13.8g; Carb: 36g; Protein: 9.4g

27. Fried Ravioli

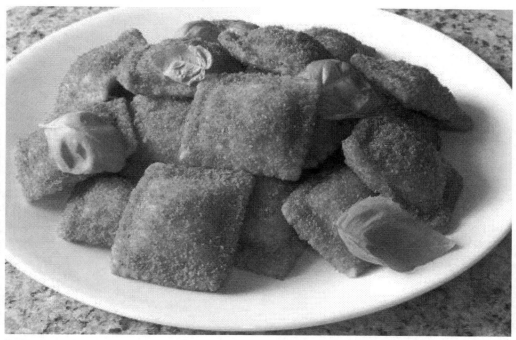

Preparation Time: 5 minutes

Cooking Time: 20 minutes

Servings: 4

Ingredients:

- 2 (9-ounce) packages frozen cheese ravioli
- 1/2 cup all-purpose flour
- 2 large eggs
- 1/2 cup milk
- 2 cups panko bread crumbs
- 1/4 cup grated Parmesan cheese
- Salt and freshly ground black pepper
- Vegetable oil, for frying

Directions:

1. Preheat the Ninja Speedi Rapid Cooker to 350 degrees F.
2. Place the ravioli in a greased 8-inch baking dish.

3. In a shallow basin, combine the flour, eggs, and milk.
4. In a separate shallow bowl, mix together the panko bread crumbs, Parmesan cheese, and salt and pepper to taste.
5. Working one at a time, dip the ravioli in the flour mixture, then the egg mixture, and finally the bread crumb mixture.
6. Place the breaded ravioli on a baking sheet.
7. Bake in the preheated Ninja Speedi Rapid Cooker for 8 minutes, or until golden brown and crispy.
8. In a large skillet over medium heat, Heat vegetable oil.
9. Fry the ravioli in the hot oil until golden brown and crispy.

Nutrition: Calories: 391kcal; Fat: 14.8g; Carb: 46g; Protein: 15.4g

28.   Baked Sweet Potato Fries

Preparation Time: 5 minutes

Cooking Time: 20 minutes

Servings: 4

Ingredients:

- 2 large sweet potatoes, cut into 1/4-inch strips
- 2 tablespoons olive oil
- 1 teaspoon garlic powder
- 1 teaspoon smoked paprika
- Salt and freshly ground black pepper

Directions:

1. Preheat the Ninja Speedi Rapid Cooker to 350 degrees F.
2. Place the sweet potato strips in a greased 8-inch baking dish.
3. Drizzle with the olive oil and sprinkle with the garlic powder, smoked paprika, and salt and pepper to taste.
4. Toss to coat. Conceal the dish with aluminum foil and bake in the preheated Ninja Speedi Rapid Cooker for 20 minutes, or until golden brown and crispy.

Nutrition: Calories: 135kcal; Fat: 6.8g; Carb: 19g; Protein: 1.4g

29.   Sweet and Sour Chicken Balls

Preparation Time: 5 minutes

Cooking Time: 20 minutes

Servings: 4

Ingredients:

- 1 pound ground chicken
- 1/4 cup panko bread crumbs

- 1/4 cup grated Parmesan cheese
- 1/4 teaspoon garlic powder
- 1/4 teaspoon onion powder
- 1/4 teaspoon dried oregano
- 2 tablespoons olive oil
- 1/2 cup sweet and sour sauce

Directions:

1. In a large basin, combine the ground chicken, bread crumbs, Parmesan, garlic powder, onion powder, and oregano until fully combined.
2. Form mixture into 1-inch balls and place them on a baking sheet lined with parchment paper.
3. Drizzle the balls with the olive oil.
4. Place the baking sheet in the Ninja Speedi Rapid Cooker and cook on high for 15 minutes.
5. Remove the baking sheet from the Ninja Speedi Rapid Cooker and pour the sweet and sour sauce over the chicken balls.
6. Return the baking sheet to the Ninja Speedi Rapid Cooker and cook for an additional 5 minutes.

Nutrition: Calories: 172kcal; Fat: 9.8g; Carb: 7g; Protein: 15.4g

30. Baked Mozzarella Sticks

Preparation Time: 5 minutes

Cooking Time: 10 minutes

Servings: 4

Ingredients:

- 1/2 cup all-purpose flour
- 2 eggs, beaten
- 1/2 cup panko bread crumbs
- 1/4 cup grated Parmesan cheese
- 1/2 teaspoon garlic powder
- 1/2 teaspoon onion powder
- 1/4 teaspoon dried oregano
- 1/4 teaspoon salt
- 1/4 teaspoon black pepper
- 12 ounces mozzarella cheese sticks
- 2 tablespoons olive oil

Directions:

1. In a shallow basin, combine the flour, eggs, bread crumbs, Parmesan, garlic powder, onion powder, oregano, salt, and pepper.
2. Dip each mozzarella cheese stick in the mixture until it is fully coated.

3. Place cheese sticks on a baking sheet lined with parchment paper.
4. Drizzle the cheese sticks with the olive oil.
5. Place the baking sheet in the Ninja Speedi Rapid Cooker and cook on high for 10 minutes.

Nutrition: Calories: 238kcal; Fat: 16.8g; Carb: 8g; Protein: 14.4g

31. Baked Potato Chips

Preparation Time: 5 minutes

Cooking Time: 20 minutes

Servings: 4

Ingredients:

- 2 large potatoes, thinly sliced
- 2 tablespoons olive oil
- 1/2 teaspoon garlic powder
- 1/2 teaspoon onion powder
- 1/4 teaspoon dried oregano
- 1/4 teaspoon salt
- 1/4 teaspoon black pepper

Directions:

1. Preheat the Ninja Speedi Rapid Cooker to 400°F.
2. Place the potato slices in a large bowl and toss with the olive oil, garlic powder, onion powder, oregano, salt, and pepper until fully coated.
3. Place the potato slices on a baking sheet lined with parchment paper.
4. Place the baking sheet in the Ninja Speedi Rapid Cooker and cook for 10 minutes.
5. Flip the chips and cook for an additional 5 minutes.

Nutrition: Calories: 121kcal; Fat: 5.8g; Carb: 17g; Protein: 2.4g

32.   Baked Kale Chips

Preparation Time: 5 minutes

Cooking Time: 20 minutes

Servings: 4

Ingredients:

- 1 bunch kale, washed and dried
- 2 tablespoons olive oil
- 1/2 teaspoon garlic powder
- 1/2 teaspoon onion powder
- 1/4 teaspoon dried oregano
- 1/4 teaspoon salt

- 1/4 teaspoon black pepper

Directions:

1. Preheat the Ninja Speedi Rapid Cooker to 350°F.
2. Place the kale in a large basin and toss with the olive oil, garlic powder, onion powder, oregano, salt, and pepper until fully coated.
3. Place the kale on a baking sheet lined with parchment paper.
4. Place the baking sheet in the Ninja Speedi Rapid Cooker and cook for 15 minutes.
5. Flip the chips and cook for an additional 5 minutes.

Nutrition: Calories: 67kcal; Fat: 5.8g; Carb: 5g; Protein: 2g

33. Baked Onion Rings

Preparation Time: 5 minutes

Cooking Time: 15 minutes

Servings: 4

Ingredients:

- 2 large onions, sliced into rings
- 1/2 cup all-purpose flour
- 2 eggs, beaten
- 1/2 cup panko bread crumbs
- 1/4 cup grated Parmesan cheese
- 1/2 teaspoon garlic powder
- 1/2 teaspoon onion powder
- 1/4 teaspoon dried oregano
- 1/4 teaspoon salt
- 1/4 teaspoon black pepper
- 2 tablespoons olive oil

Directions:

1. Preheat the Ninja Speedi Rapid Cooker to 400°F.
2. In a shallow basin, combine the flour, eggs, bread crumbs, Parmesan, garlic powder, onion powder, oregano, salt, and pepper.
3. Dip each onion ring in the mixture until it is fully coated. Place the onion rings on a baking sheet lined with parchment paper.
4. Drizzle the onion rings with the olive oil.
5. Place the baking sheet in the Ninja Speedi Rapid Cooker and cook for 10 minutes.
6. Flip the onion rings and cook for an additional 5 minutes.

Nutrition: Calories: 223kcal; Fat: 11.8g; Carb: 21g; Protein: 8.4g

34.   Baked Zucchini Rounds

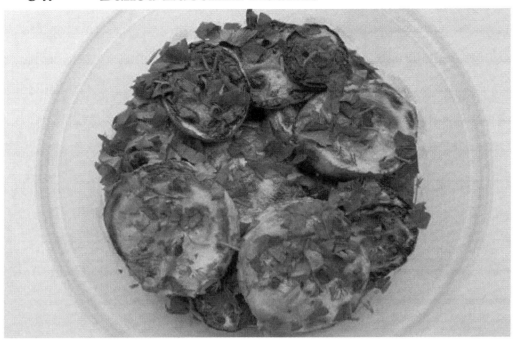

Preparation Time: 5 minutes

Cooking Time: 15 minutes

Servings: 4

Ingredients:

- 4 medium zucchini, sliced into 1/4-inch rounds
- 1/2 cup all-purpose flour
- 2 eggs, beaten
- 1/2 cup panko bread crumbs
- 1/4 cup grated Parmesan cheese
- 1/2 teaspoon garlic powder
- 1/2 teaspoon onion powder
- 1/4 teaspoon dried oregano
- 1/4 teaspoon salt
- 1/4 teaspoon black pepper
- 2 tablespoons olive oil

Directions:

1. Preheat the Ninja Speedi Rapid Cooker to 400°F.
2. In a shallow basin, combine the flour, eggs, bread crumbs, Parmesan, garlic powder, onion powder, oregano, salt, and pepper.
3. Dip each zucchini round in the mixture until it is fully coated.
4. Place zucchini rounds on a baking sheet lined with parchment paper.

5. Drizzle the zucchini rounds with the olive oil.
6. Place the baking sheet in the Ninja Speedi Rapid Cooker and cook for 10 minutes.
7. Flip the zucchini rounds and cook for an additional 5 minutes.

Nutrition: Calories: 140kcal; Fat: 8g; Carb: 10g; Protein: 6g

35.   Baked Avocado Fries

Preparation Time: 5 minutes

Cooking Time: 15 minutes

Servings: 4

Ingredients:

- 2 avocados, sliced into wedges
- 1/2 cup all-purpose flour
- 2 eggs, beaten
- 1/2 cup panko bread crumbs
- 1/4 cup grated Parmesan cheese
- 1/2 teaspoon garlic powder
- 1/2 teaspoon onion powder
- 1/4 teaspoon dried oregano
- 1/4 teaspoon salt
- 1/4 teaspoon black pepper
- 2 tablespoons olive oil

Directions:

1. Preheat the Ninja Speedi Rapid Cooker to 400°F.
2. In a shallow basin, combine the flour, eggs, bread crumbs, Parmesan, garlic powder, onion powder, oregano, salt, and pepper.
3. Dip each avocado wedge in the mixture until it is fully coated.
4. Place the avocado wedges on a baking sheet lined with parchment paper.
5. Drizzle the avocado wedges with the olive oil.
6. Place the baking sheet in the Ninja Speedi Rapid Cooker and cook for 10 minutes.
7. Flip the avocado wedges and cook for an additional 5 minutes.

Nutrition: Calories: 251kcal; Fat: 17g; Carb: 18g; Protein: 7g

36.   Baked Carrot Fries

Preparation Time: 5 minutes

Cooking Time: 20 minutes

Servings: 4

Ingredients:

- 4 large carrots, cut into 1/4-inch fries
- 2 tablespoons olive oil
- 1/2 teaspoon garlic powder
- 1/2 teaspoon onion powder
- 1/4 teaspoon dried oregano
- 1/4 teaspoon salt
- 1/4 teaspoon black pepper

Directions:

1. Preheat the Ninja Speedi Rapid Cooker to 400°F.
2. Place carrot fries in a large bowl and toss with the olive oil, garlic powder, onion powder, oregano, salt, and pepper until fully coated.
3. Place the carrot fries on a baking sheet lined with parchment paper.
4. Place the baking sheet in the Ninja Speedi Rapid Cooker and cook for 10 minutes.
5. Flip the fries and cook for an additional 5 minutes.

Nutrition: Calories: 79kcal; Fat: 5g; Carb: 8g; Protein: 1g

37.   Baked Falafel Balls

Preparation Time: 5 minutes

Cooking Time: 20 minutes

Servings: 4

Ingredients:

- 1 can chickpeas, drained and rinsed
- 1/4 cup panko bread crumbs
- 1/4 cup grated Parmesan cheese
- 1/4 teaspoon garlic powder
- 1/4 teaspoon onion powder
- 1/4 teaspoon dried oregano
- 2 tablespoons olive oil
- 1/4 cup tahini

Directions:

1. In a large bowl, combine the chickpeas, bread crumbs, Parmesan, garlic powder, onion powder, and oregano until fully combined.
2. Form mixture into 1-inch balls and place them on a baking sheet lined with parchment paper.
3. Drizzle the balls with the olive oil.
4. Place the baking sheet in the Ninja Speedi Rapid Cooker and cook on high for 15 minutes.
5. Remove the baking sheet from the Ninja Speedi Rapid Cooker and drizzle the falafel balls with the tahini.

6. Return the baking sheet to the Ninja Speedi Rapid Cooker and cook for an additional 5 minutes.

Nutrition: Calories: 171kcal; Fat: 10g; Carb: 12g; Protein: 8g

CHAPTER 3: Main Recipes

38.   Teriyaki Chicken and Broccoli

Preparation Time: 5 minutes

Cooking Time: 5 minutes

Servings: 4

Ingredients:

- 2 large boneless skinless chicken breasts, cut into cubes
- 1/2 cup teriyaki sauce
- 2 tablespoons vegetable oil
- 1/2 teaspoon ground ginger
- 2 cloves garlic, minced
- 2 cups broccoli florets
- 2 tablespoons sesame seeds
- Salt and pepper to taste

Directions:

1. Place chicken cubes in the Ninja Speedi Rapid Cooker.
2. In a small bowl, whisk together teriyaki sauce, oil, ginger, and garlic. Pour over the chicken.
3. Add the broccoli and sesame seeds. Toss to combine.
4. Cook on high for 5-6 minutes, or till chicken is cooked through.
5. Season with salt and pepper to taste. Serve over hot cooked rice.

Nutrition: Calories: 347kcal; Fat: 21g; Carb: 32g; Protein: 13g

39.   Orange Chicken

Preparation Time: 5 minutes

Cooking Time: 5-6 minutes

Servings: 4

Ingredients:

- 2 large boneless skinless chicken breasts, cut into cubes
- 1/2 cup orange marmalade
- 2 tablespoons vegetable oil
- 1 teaspoon ground ginger
- 2 cloves garlic, minced
- 1/4 cup orange juice
- 2 tablespoons cornstarch

- Salt and pepper to taste

Directions:

1. Place chicken cubes in the Ninja Speedi Rapid Cooker.
2. In a small bowl, whisk together orange marmalade, oil, ginger, garlic, orange juice, and cornstarch. Pour over the chicken.
3. Cook on high for 5-6 minutes, or till chicken is cooked through.
4. Season with salt and pepper to taste. Serve over hot cooked rice.

Nutrition: Calories: 278kcal; Fat: 7g; Carb: 32g; Protein: 25g

40.   Chicken and Rice Casserole

Preparation Time: 5 minutes

Cooking Time: 10 minutes

Servings: 4

Ingredients:

- 2 large boneless skinless chicken breasts, cut into cubes
- 2 tablespoons butter
- 1/2 cup diced onion
- 1/2 cup diced celery
- 1 cup uncooked long-grain white rice
- 2 cups chicken broth
- 1/2 teaspoon dried thyme
- 1/2 teaspoon dried oregano
- Salt and pepper to taste

Directions:

1. Place chicken cubes in the Ninja Speedi Rapid Cooker.
2. Dissolve butter in a small skillet over medium heat. Add onion and celery and sauté for 3-4 minutes.
3. Add the cooked vegetables, rice, chicken broth, thyme, and oregano to the Ninja Speedi Rapid Cooker.
4. Cook on high for 10-12 minutes, or until chicken is cooked through and rice is tender.
5. Season with salt and pepper to taste. Serve hot.

Nutrition: Calories: 354kcal; Fat: 11g; Carb: 36g; Protein: 24g

41. Chipotle Lime Shrimp

Preparation Time: 5 minutes

Cooking Time: 4-5 minutes

Servings: 4

Ingredients:

- 2 tablespoons olive oil

- 1 pound large shrimp, peeled and deveined
- 1/4 cup freshly squeezed lime juice
- 2 tbsp chipotle peppers in adobo sauce, minced
- 2 cloves garlic, minced
- 1/4 teaspoon ground cumin
- Salt and pepper to taste

Directions:

1. Place olive oil in the Ninja Speedi Rapid Cooker.
2. Add shrimp, lime juice, chipotle peppers, garlic, and cumin. Toss to combine.
3. Cook on high for 4-5 minutes, or till shrimp is cooked through.
4. Season with salt and pepper to taste. Serve over hot cooked rice.

Nutrition: Calories: 283kcal; Fat: 17g; Carb: 3g; Protein: 25g

42. Lasagna Soup

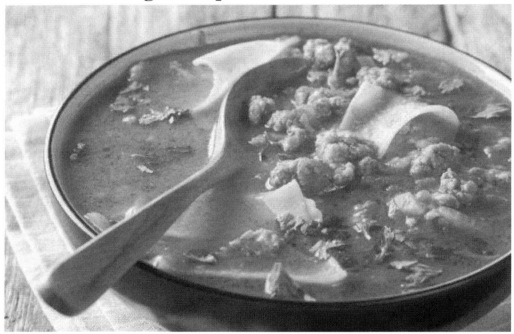

Preparation Time: 5 minutes

Cooking Time: 8 minutes

Servings: 4

Ingredients:

- 1 tablespoon olive oil
- 1 large onion, diced
- 1 clove garlic, minced
- 2 cups chicken broth

- 1 (14.5 ounce) can diced tomatoes
- 1 (15 ounce) can tomato sauce
- 4 ounces uncooked lasagna noodles, broken into pieces
- 1/2 teaspoon Italian seasoning
- 1/4 teaspoon red pepper flakes
- 2 cups baby spinach
- 1/2 cup shredded mozzarella cheese
- Salt and pepper to taste

Directions:

1. Place olive oil in the Ninja Speedi Rapid Cooker.
2. Add onion and garlic and sauté for 3-4 minutes.
3. Add chicken broth, diced tomatoes, tomato sauce, lasagna noodles, Italian seasoning, and red pepper flakes.
4. Cook on high for 8-10 minutes, or until noodles are tender.
5. Add spinach and stir to combine.
6. Add mozzarella cheese and stir until melted.
7. Season with salt and pepper to taste. Serve hot.

Nutrition: Calories: 272kcal; Fat: 7g; Carb: 38g; Protein: 16g

43.   Beef and Bean Chili

Preparation Time: 5 minutes

Cooking Time: 10-12 minutes

Servings: 4

Ingredients:

- 1 tablespoon olive oil
- 1 pound ground beef
- 1 large onion, diced
- 2 cloves garlic, minced
- 2 (14.5 ounce) cans diced tomatoes
- 2 (15 ounce) cans kidney beans, drained and washed
- 1 (4 ounce) can diced green chilies
- 1 tablespoon chili powder
- 1 teaspoon ground cumin
- 1/2 teaspoon dried oregano
- Salt and pepper to taste

Directions:

1. Place olive oil in the Ninja Speedi Rapid Cooker.

2. Add ground beef and onion and sauté for 3-4 minutes.
3. Add garlic, diced tomatoes, beans, green chilies, chili powder, cumin, and oregano.
4. Cook on high for 10-12 minutes, or until beef is cooked through.
5. Season with salt and pepper to taste. Serve over hot cooked rice.

Nutrition: Calories: 445kcal; Fat: 21g; Carb: 36g; Protein: 28g

44. Chicken Pot Pie

Preparation Time: 5 minutes

Cooking Time: 10-12 minutes

Servings: 4

Ingredients:

- 2 tablespoons butter
- 2 large boneless skinless chicken breasts, cut into cubes
- 1/2 cup diced onion
- 1/2 cup diced celery
- 1/2 cup diced carrots
- 1/2 cup frozen peas
- 1/2 cup all-purpose flour
- 2 cups chicken broth
- 1/4 cup heavy cream
- 1/2 teaspoon dried thyme
- 1/2 teaspoon dried oregano
- Salt and pepper to taste
- 2 (9 inch) unbaked pie crusts

Directions:

1. Place butter in the Ninja Speedi Rapid Cooker.
2. Add chicken, onion, celery, and carrots. Sauté for 3-4 minutes.
3. Add peas, flour, chicken broth, cream, thyme, and oregano.
4. Cook on high for 8-10 minutes, or until chicken is cooked through.
5. Place one pie crust in a 9-inch pie plate. Pour filling into the crust. Place remaining pie crust on top.
6. Cook on high for 10-12 minutes, or until crust is golden brown.
7. Season with salt and pepper to taste. Serve hot.

Nutrition: Calories: 708kcal; Fat: 40g; Carb: 56g; Protein: 28g

45. Potato and Bacon Soup

Preparation Time: 5 minutes

Cooking Time: 8-10 minutes

Servings: 4

Ingredients:

- 4 slices bacon, diced
- 1 large onion, diced
- 2 cloves garlic, minced
- 4 cups chicken broth
- 4 large potatoes, peeled and diced
- 1/2 teaspoon dried thyme
- 1/2 teaspoon dried oregano
- 1/2 cup heavy cream
- Salt and pepper to taste

Directions:

1. Place bacon in the Ninja Speedi Rapid Cooker.
2. Cook on high for 4-5 minutes, or till bacon is crisp.
3. Add onion and garlic and sauté for 3-4 minutes.
4. Add chicken broth, potatoes, thyme, and oregano.
5. Cook on high for 8-10 minutes, or until potatoes are tender.
6. Add cream and stir to combine.
7. Season with salt and pepper to taste. Serve hot.

Nutrition: Calories: 251kcal; Fat: 13g; Carb: 24g; Protein: 11g

46. Turkey Sloppy Joes

Preparation Time: 5 minutes

Cooking Time: 10 minutes

Servings: 4

Ingredients:

- 1 tablespoon olive oil
- 1 pound ground turkey
- 1 large onion, diced
- 1/2 cup ketchup
- 1/4 cup Worcestershire sauce
- 1/4 cup brown sugar
- 1 tablespoon yellow mustard
- Salt and pepper to taste
- 4 hamburger buns

Directions:

1. Place olive oil in the Ninja Speedi Rapid Cooker.

2. Add ground turkey and onion and sauté for 3-4 minutes.

3. Add ketchup, Worcestershire sauce, brown sugar, and mustard.

4. Cook on high for 8-10 minutes, or until turkey is cooked through.

5. Season with salt and pepper to taste. Serve on hamburger buns.

Nutrition: Calories: 328kcal; Fat: 13g; Carb: 31g; Protein: 22g

47.   Mango Chicken Thighs

Preparation Time: 5 minutes

Cooking Time: 5 minutes

Servings: 4

Ingredients:

- 4 boneless skinless chicken thighs
- 1/2 cup mango chutney
- 2 tablespoons honey
- 1 teaspoon curry powder
- 2 cloves garlic, minced
- Salt and pepper to taste

Directions:

1. Place chicken thighs in the Ninja Speedi Rapid Cooker.

2. In a small bowl, whisk together mango chutney, honey, curry powder, and garlic. Pour over the chicken.

3. Cook on high for 4-5 minutes, or till chicken is cooked through.

4. Season with salt and pepper to taste. Serve over hot cooked rice.

Nutrition: Calories: 426kcal; Fat: 16g; Carb: 33g; Protein: 33g

48.   Beef and Broccoli Stir-Fry

Preparation Time: 5 minutes

Cooking Time: 6 minutes

Servings: 4

Ingredients:

- beef sirloin- 1 lb., cut into thin strips
- 2 tablespoons vegetable oil
- 3 cloves garlic, minced
- 1/4 cup low-sodium soy sauce
- 2 tablespoons honey
- 2 tablespoons rice wine vinegar
- 2 tablespoons cornstarch

- 2 tablespoons water
- 2 cups broccoli florets
- 2 tablespoons toasted sesame seeds

Directions:

1. In the Ninja Speedi Rapid cooker, add the beef, vegetable oil, garlic, soy sauce, honey, and rice wine vinegar.
2. Conceal and cook on HIGH pressure for 5 minutes.
3. Quick release the pressure and open the Ninja Speedi Rapid cooker.
4. In a small bowl, whisk together the cornstarch and water.
5. Add the cornstarch mixture to the Ninja Speedi Rapid cooker and stir to combine.
6. Add the broccoli to the Ninja Speedi Rapid cooker and stir to combine.
7. Conceal and cook on HIGH pressure for 1 minute.
8. Quick release the pressure and open the Ninja Speedi Rapid cooker.
9. Sprinkle with sesame seeds and serve.

Nutrition: Calories: 318kcal; Fat: 14g; Carb: 17g; Protein: 31g

49. Thai Peanut Chicken

Preparation Time: 5 minutes

Cooking Time: 5 minutes

Servings: 4

Ingredients:

- boneless, skinless chicken breasts- 1 lb., cut into cubes
- 1/4 cup creamy peanut butter
- 1/4 cup low-sodium soy sauce
- 2 tablespoons honey
- 2 tablespoons rice wine vinegar
- 2 tablespoons sesame oil
- 1 teaspoon ground ginger
- 2 cloves garlic, minced
- 2 tablespoons green onions, thinly sliced
- 2 tablespoons chopped peanuts

Directions:

1. In the Ninja Speedi Rapid cooker, add the chicken, peanut butter, soy sauce, honey, rice wine vinegar, sesame oil, ginger, and garlic.
2. Conceal and cook on HIGH pressure for 5 minutes.
3. Quick release the pressure and open the Ninja Speedi Rapid cooker.
4. Add the green onions and stir to combine.

5. Sprinkle with peanuts and serve.

Nutrition: Calories: 292kcal; Fat: 15g; Carb: 10g; Protein: 30g

50.   Sweet and Sour Shrimp

Preparation Time: 5 minutes

Cooking Time: 3 minutes

Servings: 4

Ingredients:

- 1 lb. shrimp, peeled and deveined
- 1/4 cup ketchup
- 2 tablespoons rice vinegar
- 2 tablespoons brown sugar
- 2 tablespoons soy sauce
- 2 cloves garlic, minced
- 1/2 teaspoon red pepper flakes
- 2 tablespoons cornstarch
- 2 tablespoons water
- 1 cup pineapple chunks
- 2 tablespoons chopped cilantro

Directions:

1. In the Ninja Speedi Rapid cooker, add the shrimp, ketchup, rice vinegar, brown sugar, soy sauce, garlic and red pepper flakes.
2. Conceal and cook on HIGH pressure for 2 minutes.
3. Quick release the pressure and open the Ninja Speedi Rapid cooker.
4. In a small bowl, whisk together the cornstarch and water.
5. Add the cornstarch mixture to the Ninja Speedi Rapid cooker and stir to combine.
6. Add the pineapple chunks to the Ninja Speedi Rapid cooker and stir to combine.
7. Conceal and cook on HIGH pressure for 1 minute.
8. Quick release the pressure and open the Ninja Speedi Rapid cooker. Sprinkle with cilantro and serve.

Nutrition: Calories: 209kcal; Fat: 2g; Carb: 318g; Protein: 26g

51.Kung Pao Chicken

Preparation Time: 5 minutes

Cooking Time: 6 minutes

Servings: 4

Ingredients:

- boneless, skinless chicken breasts-1 lb., cut into cubes

- 1/4 cup low-sodium soy sauce
- 2 tablespoons rice wine vinegar
- 2 tablespoons honey
- 2 tablespoons sesame oil
- 1 teaspoon red pepper flakes
- 2 cloves garlic, minced
- 2 tablespoons cornstarch
- 2 tablespoons water
- 1/2 cup roasted peanuts
- 2 tablespoons chopped scallions

Directions:

1. In the Ninja Speedi Rapid cooker, add the chicken, soy sauce, rice wine vinegar, honey, sesame oil, red pepper flakes, and garlic.
2. Conceal and cook on HIGH pressure for 5 minutes.
3. Quick release the pressure and open the Ninja Speedi Rapid cooker.
4. In a small bowl, whisk together the cornstarch and water.
5. Add the cornstarch mixture to the Ninja Speedi Rapid cooker and stir to combine.
6. Add the peanuts to the Ninja Speedi Rapid cooker and stir to combine.
7. Conceal and cook on HIGH pressure for 1 minute.
8. Quick release the pressure and open the Ninja Speedi Rapid cooker.
9. Sprinkle with scallions and serve.

Nutrition: Calories: 334kcal; Fat: 18g; Carb: 10g; Protein: 33g

52. Orange Chicken

Preparation Time: 5 minutes

Cooking Time: 6 minutes

Servings: 4

Ingredients:

- boneless, skinless chicken breasts-1 lb. cut into cubes
- 1/2 cup orange juice
- 2 tablespoons low-sodium soy sauce
- 2 tablespoons honey
- 2 tablespoons rice wine vinegar
- 2 tablespoons sesame oil
- 2 cloves garlic, minced
- 2 tablespoons cornstarch
- 2 tablespoons water

- 1/2 cup orange segments
- 2 tablespoons toasted sesame seeds

Directions:

1. In the Ninja Speedi Rapid cooker, add the chicken, orange juice, soy sauce, honey, rice wine vinegar, sesame oil, and garlic.
2. Cover and cook on HIGH pressure for 5 minutes.
3. Quick release the pressure and open the Ninja Speedi Rapid cooker.
4. In a small bowl, whisk together the cornstarch and water.
5. Add the cornstarch mixture to the Ninja Speedi Rapid cooker and stir to combine.
6. Add the orange segments to the Ninja Speedi Rapid cooker and stir to combine.
7. Cover and cook on HIGH pressure for 1 minute.
8. Quick release the pressure and open the Ninja Speedi Rapid cooker.
9. Sprinkle with sesame seeds and serve.

Nutrition: Calories: 271kcal; Fat: 8g; Carb: 17g; Protein: 30g

53.   Coconut Curry Shrimp

Preparation Time: 5 minutes

Cooking Time: 5 minutes

Servings: 4

Ingredients:

- 1 lb. shrimp, peeled and deveined
- 1/4 cup coconut milk
- 2 tablespoons curry powder
- 1 teaspoon ground ginger
- 1/2 teaspoon ground turmeric
- 2 cloves garlic, minced
- 2 tablespoons cornstarch
- 2 tablespoons water
- 1/4 cup chopped cilantro
- 1/4 cup chopped roasted cashews

Directions:

1. In the Ninja Speedi Rapid cooker, add the shrimp, coconut milk, curry powder, ginger, turmeric, and garlic.
2. Cover and cook on HIGH pressure for 2 minutes.
3. Quick release the pressure and open the Ninja Speedi Rapid cooker.
4. In a small bowl, whisk together the cornstarch and water.
5. Add the cornstarch mixture to the Ninja Speedi Rapid cooker and stir to combine.

6. Cover and cook on HIGH pressure for 1 minute.

7. Quick release the pressure and open the Ninja Speedi Rapid cooker.

8. Sprinkle with cilantro and cashews and serve.

Nutrition: Calories: 259kcal; Fat: 9g; Carb: 9g; Protein: 29g

54.   Sesame Chicken

Preparation Time: 5 minutes

Cooking Time: 6 minutes

Servings: 4

Ingredients:

- boneless, skinless chicken breasts-1 lb. cut into cubes
- 2 tablespoons low-sodium soy sauce
- 2 tablespoons honey
- 2 tablespoons rice wine vinegar
- 2 tablespoons sesame oil
- 2 cloves garlic, minced
- 2 tablespoons cornstarch
- 2 tablespoons water
- 2 tablespoons toasted sesame seeds

Directions:

1. In the Ninja Speedi Rapid cooker, add the chicken, soy sauce, honey, rice wine vinegar, sesame oil, and garlic.

2. Cover and cook on HIGH pressure for 5 minutes.

3. Quick release the pressure and open the Ninja Speedi Rapid cooker.

4. In a small bowl, whisk together the cornstarch and water.

5. Add the cornstarch mixture to the Ninja Speedi Rapid cooker and stir to combine.

6. Cover and cook on HIGH pressure for 1 minute.

7. Quick release the pressure and open the Ninja Speedi Rapid cooker.

8. Sprinkle with sesame seeds and serve.

Nutrition: Calories: 262kcal; Fat: 9g; Carb: 9g; Protein: 33g

55.   Thai Basil Shrimp

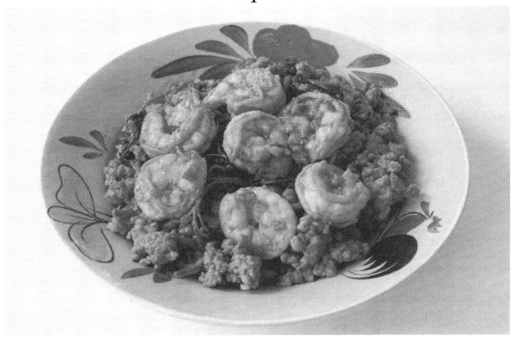

Preparation Time: 5 minutes

Cooking Time: 3 minutes

Servings: 4

Ingredients:

- 1 lb. shrimp, peeled and deveined
- 1/4 cup low-sodium soy sauce
- 2 tablespoons honey
- 2 tablespoons rice wine vinegar
- 2 tablespoons sesame oil
- 1 teaspoon red pepper flakes
- 2 cloves garlic, minced
- 2 tablespoons cornstarch
- 2 tablespoons water
- 1/4 cup chopped Thai basil
- 2 tablespoons toasted sesame seeds

Directions:

1. In the Ninja Speedi Rapid cooker, add the shrimp, soy sauce, honey, rice wine vinegar, sesame oil, red pepper flakes, and garlic.
2. Cover and cook on HIGH pressure for 2 minutes.
3. Quick release the pressure and open the Ninja Speedi Rapid cooker.
4. In a small bowl, whisk together the cornstarch and water.

5. Add the cornstarch mixture to the Ninja Speedi Rapid cooker and stir to combine.
6. Add the Thai basil to the Ninja Speedi Rapid cooker and stir to combine.
7. Cover and cook on HIGH pressure for 1 minute.
8. Quick release the pressure and open the Ninja Speedi Rapid cooker.
9. Sprinkle with sesame seeds and serve.

Nutrition: Calories: 213kcal; Fat: 8g; Carb: 9g; Protein: 25g

56.   Mongolian Beef

Preparation Time: 5 minutes

Cooking Time: 6 minutes

Servings: 4

Ingredients:

- beef sirloin- 1 lb. cut into thin strips
- 2 tablespoons vegetable oil
- 3 cloves garlic, minced
- 1/4 cup low-sodium soy sauce
- 2 tablespoons honey
- 2 tablespoons rice wine vinegar
- 2 tablespoons cornstarch
- 2 tablespoons water
- 2 tablespoons toasted sesame seeds

Directions:

1. In the Ninja Speedi Rapid cooker, add the beef, vegetable oil, garlic, soy sauce, honey, and rice wine vinegar.
2. Cover and cook on HIGH pressure for 5 minutes.
3. Quick release the pressure and open the Ninja Speedi Rapid cooker.
4. In a small bowl, whisk together the cornstarch and water.
5. Add the cornstarch mixture to the Ninja Speedi Rapid cooker and stir to combine.
6. Cover and cook on HIGH pressure for 1 minute.
7. Quick release the pressure and open the Ninja Speedi Rapid cooker.
8. Sprinkle with sesame seeds and serve.

Nutrition: Calories: 252kcal; Fat: 11g; Carb: 8g; Protein: 30g

57.   Crisp Chicken Wings

Preparation Time: 15 minutes

Cooking Time: 25 minutes

Servings: 4

Ingredients:

- ½ cup water, for steaming
- 1 pound (454 g) chicken wings
- 3 tbsps. vegetable oil
- ½ cup all-purpose flour
- ½ tsp. smoked paprika
- ½ tsp. garlic powder
- ½ tsp. kosher salt
- 1½ tsps. freshly cracked black pepper

Directions:

1. Pour ½ cup water into the pot. Push in the legs on the Crisper Tray, then place the tray in the bottom position in the pot.
2. Put the chicken wings in a large bowl. Spritz the vegetable oil over wings and toss to coat well.
3. In a separate basin, whisk together the flour, garlic powder, paprika, salt, and pepper until combined completely.
4. Dip the wings in the flour mixture one at a time, coating them well, and arrange in the tray.
5. Close and flip the SmartSwitch to Rapid Cooker. Select STEAM & CRISP, set temperature to 450°F, and set time to 25 minutes. Press START/STOP to start cooking (the unit will steam for approx. 4 minutes before crisping).
6. With 15 minutes remaining, open the lid and turn the wings over with tongs. Close the lid to continue cooking, until the breading is browned and crunchy.
7. Serve hot.

Nutrition: Calories: 289kcal; Fat: 13.8g; Carb: 26g; Protein: 9.4g

CHAPTER 4: Sides

58.   Baked Sweet Potato Slices

Preparation Time: 5 minutes

Cooking Time: 15 minutes

Servings: ½ cup

Ingredients:

- large sweet potatoes- 2, peeled and thinly sliced
- 2 tablespoons olive oil
- 1 teaspoon garlic powder
- 1 teaspoon paprika
- 1/4 teaspoon sea salt
- 1/4 teaspoon black pepper

Directions:

1. Preheat the Ninja Speedi Rapid Cooker to 350°F.
2. Place the sliced sweet potatoes in a big basin.
3. Spray with olive oil and sprinkle with garlic powder, paprika, salt and pepper.
4. Toss to coat.
5. Place the sweet potatoes in the preheated Ninja Speedi Rapid Cooker.
6. Cook for 15 minutes, stirring occasionally, until the potatoes are tender.
7. Serve warm.

Nutrition: Calories: 70kcal; Fat: 3.8g; Carb: 9g; Protein: 1g

59.   Roasted Broccoli

Preparation Time: 5 minutes

Cooking Time: 10 minutes

Servings: 4

Ingredients:

- 2 heads of broccoli, trimmed and cut into florets
- 2 tablespoons olive oil
- 1 teaspoon garlic powder
- 1/2 teaspoon paprika
- 1/4 teaspoon sea salt
- 1/4 teaspoon black pepper

Directions:

1. Preheat the Ninja Speedi Rapid Cooker to 350°F.
2. Place the broccoli florets in a large bowl.
3. Spray with olive oil and sprinkle with garlic powder, paprika, salt and pepper.
4. Toss to coat.
5. Place the broccoli in the preheated Ninja Speedi Rapid Cooker.
6. Cook for 10 minutes, stirring occasionally, until the broccoli is tender.
7. Serve warm.

Nutrition: Calories: 50kcal; Fat: 3g; Carb: 5g; Protein: 3g

60.   Garlic Parmesan Quinoa Pilaf

Preparation Time: 5 minutes

Cooking Time: 10 minutes

Servings: 4

Ingredients:

- 1 cup quinoa, rinsed
- 2 tablespoons olive oil
- 2 cloves garlic, minced
- 1/4 teaspoon sea salt
- 1/4 teaspoon black pepper
- 1/2 cup grated Parmesan cheese

Directions:

1. Preheat the Ninja Speedi Rapid Cooker to 350°F.
2. Place the quinoa in the preheated Ninja Speedi Rapid Cooker.
3. Spray with olive oil and sprinkle with garlic, salt and pepper.
4. Stir to combine.
5. Cook for 10 minutes, stirring occasionally, until the quinoa is tender.
6. Stir in the Parmesan cheese.
7. Serve warm.

Nutrition: Calories: 160kcal; Fat: 6g; Carb: 17g; Protein: 8g

61. Zucchini Fritters

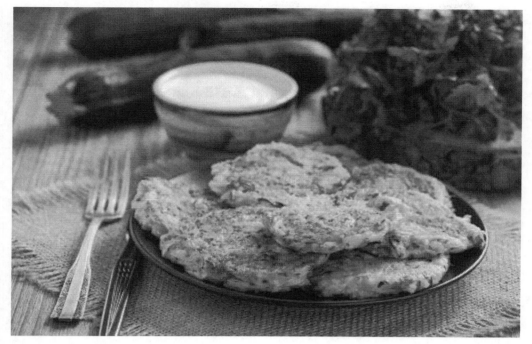

Preparation Time: 5 minutes

Cooking Time: 3 minutes

Servings: 4

Ingredients:

- 3 cups grated zucchini
- 1/2 cup shredded Cheddar cheese
- 2 large eggs, lightly beaten
- 2 tablespoons all-purpose flour
- 1/4 teaspoon sea salt
- 1/4 teaspoon black pepper
- 2 tablespoons olive oil

Directions:

1. Preheat the Ninja Speedi Rapid Cooker to 350°F.
2. Place the grated zucchini in a large bowl.
3. Add the Cheddar cheese, eggs, flour, salt and pepper.
4. Stir to combine.
5. Heat the olive oil in the preheated Ninja Speedi Rapid Cooker.
6. Drop spoonfuls of the zucchini mixture into the hot oil and press down lightly to flatten.
7. Cook for 3 minutes, flipping once, until golden brown and crispy.
8. Remove from the Ninja Speedi Rapid Cooker and serve warm.

Nutrition: Calories: 185kcal; Fat: 13g; Carb: 8g; Protein: 8g

62.   Roasted Asparagus

Preparation Time: 5 minutes

Cooking Time: 8 minutes

Servings: 4

Ingredients:

- 1 pound asparagus, trimmed
- 2 tablespoons olive oil
- 1 teaspoon garlic powder
- 1/4 teaspoon sea salt
- 1/4 teaspoon black pepper

Directions:

1. Preheat the Ninja Speedi Rapid Cooker to 350°F.
2. Place the asparagus in a large bowl.
3. Spray with olive oil and sprinkle with garlic powder, salt and pepper.
4. Toss to coat.
5. Place the asparagus in the preheated Ninja Speedi Rapid Cooker.
6. Cook for 8 minutes, stirring occasionally, until the asparagus is tender.
7. Serve warm.

Nutrition: Calories: 45kcal; Fat: 3.8g; Carb: 3g; Protein: 2g

63.   Cheesy Spinach Rice

Preparation Time: 5 minutes

Cooking Time: 15 minutes

Servings: 4

Ingredients:

- 1 cup longgrain white rice
- 1 cup chicken broth
- 2 tablespoons olive oil
- 2 cloves garlic, minced
- 3 cups fresh spinach, chopped
- 1/2 cup shredded Cheddar cheese
- 1/4 teaspoon sea salt
- 1/4 teaspoon black pepper

Directions:

1. Preheat the Ninja Speedi Rapid Cooker to 350°F.
2. Place the rice and chicken broth in the preheated Ninja Speedi Rapid Cooker.

3. Spray with olive oil and sprinkle with garlic, salt and pepper.
4. Stir to combine.
5. Cook for 10 minutes, stirring occasionally, until the rice is tender.
6. Add the chopped spinach and stir to mix.
7. Cook for another 5 minutes, stirring occasionally, until the spinach is wilted.
8. Stir in the Cheddar cheese.
9. Serve warm.

Nutrition: Calories: 160kcal; Fat: 5g; Carb: 18g; Protein: 8g

64. Greek Orzo Salad

Preparation Time: 5 minutes

Cooking Time: 15 minutes

Servings: 4

Ingredients:

- 1 cup orzo pasta
- 2 cups water
- 2 tablespoons olive oil
- 1/4 cup crumbled feta cheese
- 1/4 cup Kalamata olives, chopped
- 1/4 cup chopped fresh parsley
- 1/4 teaspoon sea salt
- 1/4 teaspoon black pepper

Directions:

1. Preheat the Ninja Speedi Rapid Cooker to 350°F.
2. Place the orzo pasta and water in the preheated Ninja Speedi Rapid Cooker.
3. Spray with olive oil and sprinkle with salt and pepper.
4. Stir to combine.
5. Cook for 10 minutes, stirring occasionally, until the orzo is tender.
6. Drain any excess liquid.
7. Stir in the feta cheese, olives and parsley.
8. Serve warm or chilled.

Nutrition: Calories: 160kcal; Fat: 5g; Carb: 21g; Protein: 5g

65. Garlic Butter Mushrooms

Preparation Time: 5 minutes

Cooking Time: 8 minutes

Servings: 4

Ingredients:

- 2 cups sliced mushrooms
- 4 tablespoons butter
- 2 cloves garlic, minced
- 1/4 teaspoon sea salt
- 1/4 teaspoon black pepper

Directions:

1. Preheat the Ninja Speedi Rapid Cooker to 350°F.
2. Place the mushrooms in the preheated Ninja Speedi Rapid Cooker.
3. Add the butter, garlic, salt and pepper.
4. Stir to combine.
5. Cook for 8 minutes, stirring occasionally, until the mushrooms are tender.
6. Serve warm.

Nutrition: Calories: 80kcal; Fat: 7g; Carb: 2g; Protein: 2g

66.   Cheesy Broccoli and Rice

Preparation Time: 5 minutes

Cooking Time: 15 minutes

Servings: 4

Ingredients:

- 1 cup long grain white rice
- 1 cup chicken broth
- 2 tablespoons olive oil
- 1 head of broccoli, trimmed and cut into florets
- 1/2 cup shredded Cheddar cheese
- 1/4 teaspoon sea salt
- 1/4 teaspoon black pepper

Directions:

1. Preheat the Ninja Speedi Rapid Cooker to 350°F.
2. Place the rice and chicken broth in the preheated Ninja Speedi Rapid Cooker.
3. Spray with olive oil and sprinkle with salt and pepper.
4. Stir to combine.
5. Cook for 10 minutes, stirring occasionally, until the rice is tender.
6. Add the broccoli and stir to combine.
7. Cook for another 5 minutes, stirring occasionally, until the broccoli is tender.
8. Stir in the Cheddar cheese.
9. Serve warm.

Nutrition: Calories: 170kcal; Fat: 6.8g; Carb: 17g; Protein: 9g

67.   Garlic Cauliflower Mash

Preparation Time: 5 minutes

Cooking Time: 15 minutes

Servings: 4

Ingredients:

- 1 head of cauliflower, cut into florets
- 1/4 cup chicken broth
- 2 cloves garlic, minced
- 3 tablespoons butter
- 1/4 teaspoon sea salt
- 1/4 teaspoon black pepper

Directions:

1. Preheat the Ninja Speedi Rapid Cooker to 350°F.
2. Place the cauliflower florets in the preheated Ninja Speedi Rapid Cooker.
3. Add the chicken broth, garlic, butter, salt and pepper.
4. Stir to combine.
5. Cook for 8 minutes, stirring occasionally, until the cauliflower is tender.
6. Mash with a potato masher or blend in a blender until smooth.
7. Serve warm.

Nutrition: Calories: 70kcal; Fat: 5g; Carb: 5g; Protein: 2g

CHAPTER 5: Soup and Salad

68.   Spicy Chicken Tortilla Soup

Preparation Time: 5 minutes

Cooking Time: 20 minutes

Servings: 4

Ingredients:

- 1 tablespoon olive oil
- 2 cloves garlic, minced
- 1/2 cup diced onion
- 1 teaspoon ground cumin
- 1/2 teaspoon chili powder
- 1/4 teaspoon salt
- 1/4 teaspoon freshly ground black pepper
- 1 (14.5-ounce) can diced tomatoes
- 2 cups chicken broth
- boneless, skinless chicken breasts- 2, cut into cubes
- black beans- 1 (15-ounce) can, drained and rinsed
- 1 cup frozen corn
- 1/4 cup chopped fresh cilantro
- 1/4 cup chopped fresh parsley
- 2 tablespoons fresh lime juice
- 3 (6-inch) corn tortillas, cut into strips

Directions:

1. Heat the oil in the Ninja Speedi Rapid Cooker over medium heat.
2. Add the garlic, onion, cumin, chili powder, salt, and pepper. Cook, stirring often, until the onion is soft, about 5 minutes.
3. Add the tomatoes, chicken broth, chicken, black beans, corn, cilantro, and parsley. Stir to combine.
4. Close and seal the lid. Cook on high pressure for 15 minutes.
5. Release the pressure making use of the quick release method. Open the lid and stir in the lime juice.
6. Place the tortilla strips in the soup and stir to combine. Cook for an additional 5 minutes.
7. Serve the soup with extra tortilla strips and garnish with extra cilantro and parsley, if desired.

Nutrition: Calories: 288kcal; Fat: 5g; Carb: 34g; Protein: 22.4g

69. Creamy Mushroom Soup

Preparation Time: 5 minutes

Cooking Time: 15 minutes

Servings: 4

Ingredients:

- 1 tablespoon butter
- 1/2 cup chopped onion
- 1/2 teaspoon garlic powder
- 2 cups sliced mushrooms
- 1/4 teaspoon dried thyme
- 2 tablespoons all-purpose flour
- 4 cups chicken broth
- 1 cup half-and-half
- 1/4 teaspoon freshly ground black pepper
- 1/4 teaspoon freshly ground nutmeg
- 2 tablespoons chopped fresh parsley

Directions:

1. Heat the butter in the Ninja Speedi Rapid Cooker over medium heat.
2. Add the onion, garlic powder, mushrooms, and thyme. Cook, stirring often, until the onion is soft, about 5 minutes.
3. Add the flour and stir until combined.
4. Add the chicken broth and stir until combined.
5. Close and seal the lid. Cook on high pressure for 10 minutes.
6. Release the pressure utilizing the quick release method. Open the lid and stir in the half-and-half.
7. Cook for an additional 5 minutes.
8. Stir in the pepper, nutmeg, and parsley.
9. Serve the soup with extra parsley for garnish, if desired.

Nutrition: Calories: 148kcal; Fat: 8g; Carb: 16g; Protein: 6.4g

70. Hearty Minestrone Soup

Preparation Time: 5 minutes

Cooking Time: 15 minutes

Servings: 4

Ingredients:

- 1 tablespoon olive oil
- 1/2 cup chopped onion

- 3 cloves garlic, minced
- 1 teaspoon dried oregano
- 1/2 teaspoon dried basil
- 1/4 teaspoon dried thyme
- 1 (14-ounce) can diced tomatoes
- 3 cups chicken broth
- 1 (15-ounce) can kidney beans, drained and rinsed
- 1 (15-ounce) can white beans, drained and rinsed
- 1 cup small pasta shells
- 1 cup chopped carrots
- 1/2 cup frozen peas
- 1/4 cup chopped fresh parsley

Directions:

1. Heat the oil in the Ninja Speedi Rapid Cooker over medium heat.
2. Add the onion, garlic, oregano, basil, and thyme. Cook, stirring often, until the onion is soft, about 5 minutes.
3. Add the tomatoes, chicken broth, kidney beans, white beans, pasta, carrots, and peas. Stir to combine.
4. Close and seal the lid. Cook on high pressure for 10 minutes.
5. Release the pressure utilizing the quick release method. Open the lid and stir in the parsley.
6. Serve the soup with extra parsley for garnish, if desired.

Nutrition: Calories: 298kcal; Fat: 4.8g; Carb: 46g; Protein: 14.4g

71. Mediterranean Lentil Soup

Preparation Time: 5 minutes

Cooking Time: 20 minutes

Servings: 4

Ingredients:

- 1 tablespoon olive oil
- 1/2 cup diced onion
- 1 large carrot, diced
- 3 cloves garlic, minced
- 1 teaspoon ground cumin
- 1/4 teaspoon ground coriander
- 1/4 teaspoon ground turmeric
- 1 (14.5-ounce) can diced tomatoes
- 4 cups vegetable broth
- 1 cup dried lentils

- 1/4 cup chopped fresh parsley
- 1/4 cup chopped fresh cilantro
- 2 tablespoons fresh lemon juice

Directions:

1. Heat the oil in the Ninja Speedi Rapid Cooker over medium heat.
2. Add the onion, carrot, garlic, cumin, coriander, and turmeric. Cook, stirring often, until the onion is soft, about 5 minutes.
3. Add the tomatoes, vegetable broth, and lentils. Stir to combine.
4. Close and seal the lid. Cook on high pressure for 15 minutes.
5. Release the pressure utilizing the quick release method. Open the lid and stir in the parsley, cilantro, and lemon juice.
6. Serve the soup with extra parsley and cilantro for garnish, if desired.

Nutrition: Calories: 254kcal; Fat: 4.8g; Carb: 36g; Protein: 13.4g

72.   Taco Soup

Preparation Time: 5 minutes

Cooking Time: 15 minutes

Servings: 4

Ingredients:

- 1 tablespoon olive oil
- 1/2 cup diced onion
- 1 teaspoon chili powder
- 1/2 teaspoon ground cumin
- 1/4 teaspoon garlic powder
- 1/4 teaspoon salt
- 1/4 teaspoon freshly ground black pepper
- 1 (14.5-ounce) can diced tomatoes
- 1 (15-ounce) can black beans, drained and cleaned
- 1 (15-ounce) can pinto beans, drained and rinsed
- 2 cups chicken broth
- 1 cup frozen corn
- 1/4 cup chopped fresh cilantro
- 2 tablespoons fresh lime juice
- 3 (6-inch) corn tortillas, cut into strips

Directions:

1. Heat the oil in the Ninja Speedi Rapid Cooker over medium heat.

2. Add the onion, chili powder, cumin, garlic powder, salt, and pepper. Cook, stirring often, until the onion is soft, about 5 minutes.

3. Add the tomatoes, black beans, pinto beans, chicken broth, corn, and cilantro. Stir to combine.

4. Close and seal the lid. Cook on high pressure for 10 minutes.

5. Release the pressure utilizing the quick release method. Open the lid and stir in the lime juice.

6. Place the tortilla strips in the soup and stir to combine. Cook for an additional 5 minutes.

7. Serve the soup with extra tortilla strips and garnish with extra cilantro, if desired.

Nutrition: Calories: 317kcal; Fat: 6.8g; Carb: 45g; Protein: 18.4g

73. Chicken Noodle Soup

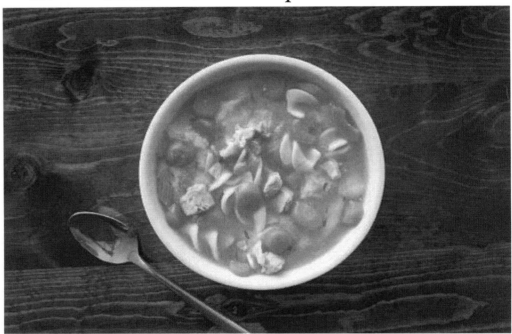

Preparation Time: 5 minutes

Cooking Time: 15 minutes

Servings: 4

Ingredients:

- 1 tablespoon olive oil
- 1/2 cup diced onion
- 2 cloves garlic, minced
- 2 cups chicken broth
- 2 cups water
- boneless, skinless chicken breasts- 2, cut into cubes
- 2 tablespoons fresh parsley, chopped
- 1/4 teaspoon freshly ground black pepper

- 1/4 teaspoon salt
- 2 cups egg noodles

Directions:

1. Heat the oil in the Ninja Speedi Rapid Cooker over medium heat.
2. Add the onion and garlic. Cook, stirring often, until the onion is soft, about 5 minutes.
3. Add the broth, water, chicken, parsley, pepper, and salt. Stir to combine.
4. Close and seal the lid. Cook on high pressure for 10 minutes.
5. Release the pressure utilizing the quick release method. Open the lid and stir in the egg noodles.
6. Cook for an additional 5 minutes.
7. Serve the soup with extra parsley for garnish, if desired.

Nutrition: Calories: 267kcal; Fat: 6.8g; Carb: 24g; Protein: 25.4g

74. Creamy Tomato Soup

Preparation Time: 5 minutes

Cooking Time: 15 minutes

Servings: 4

Ingredients:

- 1 tablespoon butter
- 1/2 cup chopped onion
- 2 cloves garlic, minced
- 1 teaspoon dried oregano
- 1 (14.5-ounce) can diced tomatoes
- 4 cups chicken broth
- 1/4 teaspoon freshly ground black pepper
- 1/4 teaspoon freshly ground nutmeg
- 1 cup half-and-half
- 2 tablespoons chopped fresh parsley

Directions:

1. Heat the butter in the Ninja Speedi Rapid Cooker over medium heat.
2. Add the onion, garlic, and oregano. Cook, stirring often, until the onion is soft, about 5 minutes.
3. Add the tomatoes and chicken broth. Stir to combine.
4. Close and seal the lid. Cook on high pressure for 10 minutes.
5. Release the pressure utilizing the quick release method. Open the lid and stir in the pepper, nutmeg, and half-and-half.
6. Cook for an additional 5 minutes.
7. Stir in the parsley.
8. Serve the soup with extra parsley for garnish, if desired.

Nutrition: Calories: 202kcal; Fat: 9.8g; Carb: 16g; Protein: 10.4g

75. Curried Butternut Squash Soup

Preparation Time: 5 minutes

Cooking Time: 20 minutes

Servings: 4

Ingredients:

- 1 tablespoon butter
- 1/2 cup chopped onion
- 1 teaspoon curry powder
- 1/2 teaspoon ground cumin
- 1/4 teaspoon ground cardamom
- 1 (14.5-ounce) can diced tomatoes
- 4 cups vegetable broth
- 1 small butternut squash, skinned, seeded, and cubed
- 1/4 teaspoon freshly ground black pepper
- 1/4 teaspoon freshly ground nutmeg
- 2 tablespoons chopped fresh parsley

Directions:

1. Heat the butter in the Ninja Speedi Rapid Cooker over medium heat.
2. Add the onion, curry powder, cumin, and cardamom. Cook, stirring often, until the onion is soft, about 5 minutes.
3. Add the tomatoes, vegetable broth, butternut squash, pepper, and nutmeg. Stir to combine.
4. Close and seal the lid. Cook on high pressure for 15 minutes.
5. Release the pressure utilizing the quick release method. Open the lid and stir in the parsley.
6. Serve the soup with extra parsley for garnish, if desired.

Nutrition: Calories: 155kcal; Fat: 4.8g; Carb: 26g; Protein: 4.4g

76. Broccoli Cheese Soup

Preparation Time: 5 minutes

Cooking Time: 15 minutes

Servings: 4

Ingredients:

- 1 tablespoon butter
- 1/2 cup chopped onion
- 2 cloves garlic, minced
- 4 cups chicken broth

- 2 cups broccoli florets
- 1/4 teaspoon freshly ground black pepper
- 1/4 teaspoon freshly ground nutmeg
- 1 cup shredded cheddar cheese
- 2 tablespoons chopped fresh parsley

Directions:

1. Heat the butter in the Ninja Speedi Rapid Cooker over medium heat.
2. Add the onion and garlic. Cook, stirring often, until the onion is soft, about 5 minutes.
3. Add the chicken broth, broccoli, pepper, and nutmeg. Stir to combine.
4. Close and seal the lid. Cook on high pressure for 10 minutes.
5. Release the pressure using quick release method. Open the lid and stir in the cheese.
6. Cook for an additional 5 minutes.
7. Stir in the parsley.
8. Serve the soup with extra parsley for garnish, if desired.

Nutrition: Calories: 211kcal; Fat: 12.8g; Carb: 10g; Protein: 17.4g

77.   Split Pea Soup

Preparation Time: 5 minutes

Cooking Time: 25 minutes

Servings: 4

Ingredients:

- 1 tablespoon olive oil
- 1/2 cup chopped onion
- 3 cloves garlic, minced
- 1 teaspoon dried oregano
- 1/2 teaspoon dried basil
- 1/4 teaspoon dried thyme
- 1 (14.5-ounce) can diced tomatoes
- 4 cups chicken broth
- 1 cup dried split peas
- 1/4 cup chopped fresh parsley
- 1/4 cup chopped fresh cilantro
- 2 tablespoons fresh lemon juice

Directions:

1. Heat the oil in the Ninja Speedi Rapid Cooker over medium heat.
2. Add the onion, garlic, oregano, basil, and thyme. Cook, stirring often, until the onion is soft, about 5 minutes.

3. Add the tomatoes, chicken broth, and split peas. Stir to combine.
4. Close and seal the lid. Cook on high pressure for 20 minutes.
5. Release the pressure using quick release method. Open the lid and stir in the parsley, cilantro, and lemon juice.
6. Serve the soup with extra parsley and cilantro for garnish, if desired.

Nutrition: Calories: 295kcal; Fat: 5.8g; Carb: 37g; Protein: 18.4g

78. Chicken Caesar Salad

Preparation Time: 5 minutes

Cooking Time: 15 minutes

Servings: 4

Ingredients:

- 2 boneless, skinless chicken breasts
- 2 tablespoons olive oil
- 2 tablespoons red wine vinegar
- 2 tablespoons grated Parmesan cheese
- 1 head romaine lettuce, chopped
- 1/4 cup croutons
- 1/4 cup shredded mozzarella cheese
- Salt and pepper to taste

Directions:

1. Place the chicken breasts in the Ninja Speedi Rapid Cooker and pour in the olive oil.
2. Cook on high for 10 minutes.
3. Remove the chicken from the pot and shred it with two forks.
4. In a large basin, combine the shredded chicken, red wine vinegar, Parmesan cheese, romaine lettuce, croutons and mozzarella cheese.
5. Mix until all ingredients are evenly distributed.
6. Add salt and pepper to taste.
7. Place the salad in the Ninja Speedi Rapid Cooker and cook on high for 5 minutes.
8. Serve the salad immediately.

Nutrition: Calories: 380kcal; Fat: 22g; Carb: 12g; Protein: 29g

79.   Greek Salad

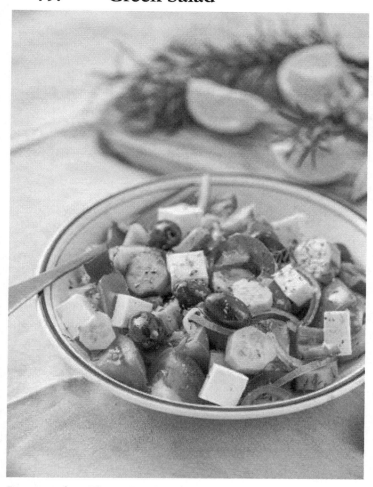

Preparation Time: 5 minutes

Cooking Time: 10 minutes

Servings: 4

Ingredients:

- 2 cups cooked quinoa
- 1 cup cherry tomatoes, halved
- 1/2 cup kalamata olives, halved
- 1/2 cup cucumber, diced
- 1/4 cup feta cheese
- 2 tablespoons olive oil
- 2 tablespoons red wine vinegar
- Salt and pepper to taste

Directions:

1.   Place the cooked quinoa in the Ninja Speedi Rapid Cooker.
2.   Add the cherry tomatoes, olives, cucumber, feta cheese, olive oil and red wine vinegar.

3. Mix until all ingredients are evenly distributed.
4. Add salt and pepper to taste.
5. Cook on high for 10 minutes.
6. Serve the salad immediately.

Nutrition: Calories: 350kcal; Fat: 16.8g; Carb: 35g; Protein: 14g

80.   Taco Salad

Preparation Time: 5 minutes

Cooking Time: 20 minutes

Servings: 4

Ingredients:

- 1 pound ground beef
- 1/2 cup salsa
- 1/4 cup taco seasoning
- 1 head romaine lettuce, chopped
- 1/2 cup corn
- 1/2 cup black beans
- 1/2 cup shredded cheddar cheese
- 1/4 cup sour cream
- 1/4 cup diced tomatoes
- 1/4 cup sliced black olives
- Salt and pepper to taste

Directions:

1. Place the ground beef in the Ninja Speedi Rapid Cooker and cook on high for 10 minutes.
2. Add the salsa and taco seasoning and mix until the beef is evenly coated.
3. Add the remaining ingredients and mix until all ingredients are evenly distributed.
4. Add salt and pepper to taste.
5. Cook on high for 10 minutes.
6. Serve the salad immediately.

Nutrition: Calories: 420kcal; Fat: 24.8g; Carb: 21g; Protein: 32g

81.Cobb Salad

Preparation Time: 5 minutes

Cooking Time: 15 minutes

Servings: 4

Ingredients:

- 2 boneless, skinless chicken breasts

- 2 tablespoons olive oil
- 2 tablespoons red wine vinegar
- 1 head romaine lettuce, chopped
- 4 slices cooked bacon, crumbled
- 1/4 cup crumbled blue cheese
- 1/4 cup diced tomatoes
- 1/4 cup diced red onion
- 1/4 cup sliced hardboiled eggs
- Salt and pepper to taste

Directions:

1. Place the chicken breasts in the Ninja Speedi Rapid Cooker and pour in the olive oil.
2. Cook on high for 10 minutes.
3. Remove the chicken from the pot and shred it with two forks.
4. In a large basin, combine the shredded chicken, red wine vinegar, romaine lettuce, bacon, blue cheese, tomatoes, red onion and eggs.
5. Mix until all ingredients are evenly distributed.
6. Add salt and pepper to taste.
7. Place the salad in the Ninja Speedi Rapid Cooker and cook on high for 5 minutes.
8. Serve the salad immediately.

Nutrition: Calories: 360kcal; Fat: 24.8g; Carb: 9g; Protein: 28g

82.　　Mediterranean Salad

Preparation Time: 5 minutes

Cooking Time: 10 minutes

Servings: 4

Ingredients:

- 2 cups cooked quinoa
- 1/2 cup canned chickpeas, drained and rinsed
- 1/2 cup diced red onion
- 1/2 cup diced cucumber
- 1/4 cup diced tomatoes
- 1/4 cup sliced kalamata olives
- 2 tablespoons olive oil
- 2 tablespoons red wine vinegar
- Salt and pepper to taste

Directions:

1. Place the cooked quinoa in the Ninja Speedi Rapid Cooker.

2. Add the chickpeas, red onion, cucumber, tomatoes, olives, olive oil and red wine vinegar.

3. Mix until all ingredients are evenly distributed.

4. Add salt and pepper to taste.

5. Cook on high for 10 minutes.

6. Serve the salad immediately.

Nutrition: Calories: 360kcal; Fat: 14.8g; Carb: 42g; Protein: 12g

83.　　Pasta Salad

Preparation Time: 5 minutes

Cooking Time: 10 minutes

Servings: 4

Ingredients:

- 2 cups cooked rotini pasta
- 1/2 cup cherry tomatoes, halved
- 1/2 cup diced cucumber
- 1/2 cup diced red onion
- 1/4 cup sliced black olives
- 2 tablespoons olive oil
- 2 tablespoons red wine vinegar
- Salt and pepper to taste

Directions:

1. Place the cooked pasta in the Ninja Speedi Rapid Cooker.

2. Add the cherry tomatoes, cucumber, red onion, olives, olive oil and red wine vinegar.

3. Mix until all ingredients are evenly distributed.

4. Add salt and pepper to taste.

5. Cook on high for 10 minutes.

6. Serve the salad immediately.

Nutrition: Calories: 360kcal; Fat: 14g; Carb: 48g; Protein: 9g

84.　　Broccoli Salad

Preparation Time: 5 minutes

Cooking Time: 10 minutes

Servings: 4

Ingredients:

- 2 cups cooked broccoli florets
- 1/2 cup diced red onion
- 1/2 cup raisins

- 1/4 cup sunflower seeds
- 2 tablespoons honey
- 2 tablespoons olive oil
- 2 tablespoons red wine vinegar
- Salt and pepper to taste

Directions:

1. Place the cooked broccoli florets in the Ninja Speedi Rapid Cooker.
2. Add the red onion, raisins, sunflower seeds, honey, olive oil and red wine vinegar.
3. Mix until all ingredients are evenly distributed.
4. Add salt and pepper to taste.
5. Cook on high for 10 minutes.
6. Serve the salad immediately.

Nutrition: Calories: 280kcal; Fat: 14g; Carb: 34g; Protein: 8g

85.   Quinoa Salad

Preparation Time: 5 minutes

Cooking Time: 10 minutes

Servings: 4

Ingredients:

- 2 cups cooked quinoa
- 1/2 cup diced carrots
- 1/2 cup diced red bell pepper
- 1/2 cup diced celery
- 1/4 cup sliced almonds
- 2 tablespoons olive oil
- 2 tablespoons balsamic vinegar
- Salt and pepper to taste

Directions:

1. Place the cooked quinoa in the Ninja Speedi Rapid Cooker.
2. Add the carrots, bell pepper, celery, almonds, olive oil and balsamic vinegar.
3. Mix until all ingredients are evenly distributed.
4. Add salt and pepper to taste.
5. Cook on high for 10 minutes.
6. Serve the salad immediately.

Nutrition: Calories: 320kcal; Fat: 16g; Carb: 33g; Protein: 8g

86.   Kale Salad

Preparation Time: 5 minutes

Cooking Time: 10 minutes

Servings: 4

Ingredients:

- 2 cups chopped kale
- 1/2 cup diced red onion
- 1/2 cup diced apples
- 1/4 cup dried cranberries
- 2 tablespoons olive oil
- 2 tablespoons balsamic vinegar
- Salt and pepper to taste

Directions:

1. Place the chopped kale in the Ninja Speedi Rapid Cooker.
2. Add the red onion, apples, cranberries, olive oil and balsamic vinegar.
3. Mix until all ingredients are evenly distributed.
4. Add salt and pepper to taste.
5. Cook on high for 10 minutes.
6. Serve the salad immediately.

Nutrition: Calories: 220kcal; Fat: 10g; Carb: 28g; Protein: 5g

87.   Spinach Salad

Preparation Time: 5 minutes

Cooking Time: 10 minutes

Servings: 4

Ingredients:

- 2 cups chopped spinach
- 1/2 cup diced red onion
- 1/2 cup dried cranberries
- 1/4 cup sliced almonds
- 2 tablespoons olive oil
- 2 tablespoons balsamic vinegar
- Salt and pepper to taste

Directions:

1. Place the chopped spinach in the Ninja Speedi Rapid Cooker.
2. Add the red onion, cranberries, almonds, olive oil and balsamic vinegar.

3. Mix until all ingredients are evenly distributed.
4. Add salt and pepper to taste.
5. Cook on high for 10 minutes.
6. Serve the salad immediately.

Nutrition: Calories: 200kcal; Fat: 10g; Carb: 22g; Protein: 4g

CHAPTER 6: Vegetables

88.   Russet Potato Gratin

Preparation Time: 10 minutes

Cooking Time: 25 minutes

Servings: 6

Ingredients:

- ½ cup water, for steaming
- ½ cup milk
- 7 medium russet potatoes, peeled
- Salt, to taste
- 1 tsp. black pepper
- ½ cup heavy whipping cream
- ½ cup grated semimature cheese
- ½ tsp. nutmeg

Directions:

1. Pour ½ cup water into the pot. Push in the legs on the Crisper Tray, then place the tray in the bottom position in the pot.
2. Slice the potatoes into waferthin slices.
3. In a bowl, mix the milk and cream and sprinkle with salt, pepper, and nutmeg.
4. Pour the milk mixture to coat the slices of potatoes. Put in a 8inch round baking pan and top the potatoes with the rest of the milk mixture. Transfer the pan to the tray.
5. Close and flip the SmartSwitch to Rapid Cooker. Select STEAM & CRISP, set temperature to 450°F, and set time to 25 minutes. Press START/STOP to start cooking (the unit will steam for approx. 10 minutes before crisping).
6. Add the cheese over the potatoes.
7. Bake for another 10 minutes, ensuring the top is nicely browned before serving.

Nutrition: Calories: 288kcal; Fat: 13.8g; Carb: 36g; Protein: 9.4g

89.   Lush Vegetables Roast

Preparation Time: 15 minutes

Cooking Time: 17 minutes

Servings: 6

Ingredients:

- 1⅓ cups small parsnips, peeled and cubed

- 1⅓ cups celery
- 2 red onions, sliced
- 1⅓ cups small butternut squash, cut in half, deseeded and cubed
- 1 tbsp. fresh thyme needles
- 1 tbsp. olive oil
- Salt and ground black pepper, to taste

Directions:

1. Push in the legs on the Crisper Tray, then place the tray in the bottom of the pot. Spray the tray with cooking spray.
2. Combine the cut vegetables with the thyme, olive oil, salt and pepper.
3. Close and flip the SmartSwitch to AIRFRY/STOVETOP. Select BAKE&ROAST, set temperature to 390°F, and set time to 22 minutes (unit will need to preheat for 5 minutes, so set an external timer if desired). Press START/STOP to start cooking.
4. When the unit is preheated and the time reaches 17 minutes, place the vegetables on the tray. Close the lid to begin cooking.
5. After 10 minutes, open the lid and toss the vegetables with silicone tipped tongs to ensure even cooking. Close the lid to continue cooking.
6. When cooking is complete, serve warm.

Nutrition: Calories: 230kcal; Fat: 3g; Carb: 2g; Protein: 9g

90. Ratatouille

Preparation Time: 20 minutes

Cooking Time: 22 minutes

Servings: 4

Ingredients:

- cooking spray
- 1 sprig basil
- 1 sprig flatleaf parsley
- 1 sprig mint
- 1 tbsp. coriander powder
- 1 tsp. capers
- ½ lemon, juiced
- 2 eggplants, sliced crosswise
- 2 red onions, chopped
- 4 cloves garlic, minced
- 5 tbsps. olive oil
- 2 red peppers, chopped

- 1 fennel bulb, sliced crosswise
- 3 large zucchinis, sliced crosswise
- 4 large tomatoes, sliced crosswise
- 2 tsps. herbs de Provence
- Salt and ground black pepper, to taste

Directions:

1. Push in the legs on the Crisper Tray, then place the tray in the bottom of the pot. Spray a 8inch round baking pan with cooking spray.
2. Blend the basil, parsley, coriander, mint, lemon juice and capers, with a pinch of salt and pepper. Ensure the ingredients are well incorporated.
3. Coat the eggplant, onions, peppers, fennel, garlic, and zucchini with olive oil.
4. Close and flip the SmartSwitch to AIRFRY/STOVETOP. Select AIRFRY, set temperature to 390°F, and set time to 27 minutes (unit will need to preheat for 5 minutes, so set an external timer if desired). Press START/STOP to begin cooking.
5. When the unit is preheated and the time reaches 22 minutes, place the vegetables in the pan, then transfer to the tray. Top with the tomatoes and herb purée. Season with more salt and pepper, and the herbs de Provence. Close the lid to begin cooking.
6. After 10 minutes, open the lid and toss the vegetables with silicone tipped tongs to ensure even cooking. Close the lid to continue cooking.
7. When cooking is complete, serve immediately.

Nutrition: Calories: 230kcal; Fat: 2g; Carb: 2g; Protein: 10g

91.Super Vegetable Burger

Preparation Time: 15 minutes

Cooking Time: 16 minutes

Servings: 8

Ingredients:

- 1 cup water, for steaming
- ½ pound (227 g) cauliflower, steamed and diced, rinsed and drained
- 1 cup bread crumbs
- ¼ cup desiccated coconut
- ½ cup oats
- 2 tsps. coconut oil, melted
- 2 tsps. minced garlic
- 3 tbsps. flour
- 1 tbsp. flaxseeds plus 3 tbsps. water, divided
- 1 tsp. mustard powder

- 2 tsps. thyme
- 2 tsps. parsley
- 2 tsps. chives
- Salt and ground black pepper, to taste

Directions:

1. Pour 1 cup water into the pot. Push in the legs on the Crisper Tray, then place the tray in the bottom position in the pot.
2. Mix all the ingredients, except for the bread crumbs, incorporating everything well.
3. Using the hands, form 8 equal sized amounts of the mixture into burger patties. Coat the patties in bread crumbs before putting them to the tray in a single layer.
4. Close and flip the SmartSwitch to Rapid Cooker. Select STEAM & CRISP, set temperature to 390°F, and set time to 12 minutes. Press START/STOP to start cooking (the unit will steam for approx. 4 minutes before crisping).
5. With 6 minutes remaining, open the lid and flip the burgers with tongs. Close the lid to continue cooking.
6. When cooking is complete, use tongs to remove the burgers from the tray and serve hot.

Nutrition: Calories: 130kcal; Fat: 3g; Carb: 2g; Protein: 6g

92.   Balsamic Brussels Sprouts

Preparation Time: 5 minutes

Cooking Time: 15 minutes

Servings: 2

Ingredients:

- ½ cup water, for steaming
- 2 cups Brussels sprouts, halved
- 1 tbsp. olive oil
- 1 tbsp. balsamic vinegar
- 1 tbsp. maple syrup
- ¼ tsp. sea salt

Directions:

1. Pour ½ cup water into the pot. Push in the legs on the Crisper Tray, then place the tray in the bottom position in the pot.
2. Coat the Brussels sprouts well with the olive oil, balsamic vinegar, maple syrup, and salt. Transfer the Brussels sprouts to the tray.
3. Close and flip the SmartSwitch to Rapid Cooker. Select STEAM & CRISP, set temperature to 450°F, and set time to 15 minutes. Press START/STOP to start cooking (the unit will steam for approx. 4 minutes before crisping).

4. With 10 minutes remaining, open the lid and toss the Brussels sprouts with tongs. Close the lid to continue cooking. Repeat this process when 5 minutes remain.
5. When cooking is complete, use tongs to remove the Brussels sprouts from the tray and serve hot.

Nutrition: Calories: 212kcal; Fat: 2g; Carb: 3g; Protein: 9g

93.   Sweet Potatoes with Tofu

Preparation Time: 15 minutes

Cooking Time: 29 minutes

Servings: 8

Ingredients:

- ½ cup water, for steaming
- 8 sweet potatoes, scrubbed
- 2 tbsps. olive oil
- 1 large onion, chopped
- 2 green chilies, deseeded and chopped
- 8 ounces (227 g) tofu, crumbled
- 2 tbsps. Cajun seasoning
- 1 cup chopped tomatoes
- 1 can kidney beans, drained and rinsed
- Salt and ground black pepper, to taste

Directions:

1. Pour ½ cup water into the pot. Push in the legs on the Crisper Tray, then place the tray in the bottom position in the pot.
2. Pierce the skin of the sweet potatoes with a knife, then transfer to the tray.
3. Close and flip the SmartSwitch to Rapid Cooker. Select STEAM & CRISP, set temperature to 450°F, and set time to 22 minutes. Press START/STOP to start cooking (the unit will steam for approx. 4 minutes before crisping).
4. With 15 minutes remaining, open the lid and toss the sweet potatoes with tongs. Close the lid to continue cooking. Repeat this process when 5 minutes remain.
5. When the sweet potatoes are cooking, fry the onions and chilies in the olive oil in a skillet over a medium heat, for 2 minutes until fragrant.
6. When the cook of sweet potatoes is finished, halve each potato, and set to one side.
7. Place the tofu and Cajun seasoning to the tray and cook for a further 3 minutes before incorporating the kidney beans and tomatoes. Season with some salt and pepper as desire.
8. Top each sweet potato halve with a spoonful of the tofu mixture and serve warm.

Nutrition: Calories: 189kcal; Fat: 3g; Carb: 2g; Protein: 10g

94.   Rice and Eggplant Bowl

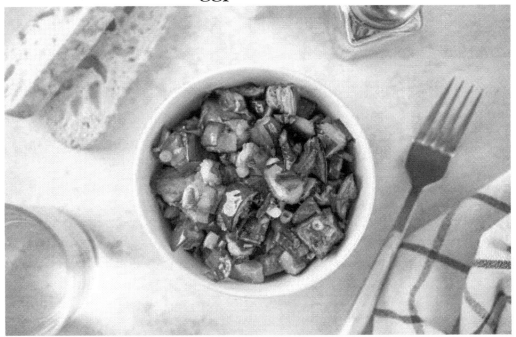

Preparation Time: 15 minutes

Cooking Time: 10 minutes

Servings: 4

Ingredients:

- ¼ cup sliced cucumber
- 1 tsp. salt
- 1 tbsp. sugar
- 7 tbsps. Japanese rice vinegar
- 3 medium eggplants, sliced
- 3 tbsps. sweet white miso paste
- 1 tbsp. mirin rice wine
- 4 cups cooked sushi rice
- 4 spring onions
- 1 tbsp. toasted sesame seeds

Directions:

1. Push in the legs on the Crisper Tray, then place the tray in the bottom of the pot. Spray the tray with cooking spray.
2. In a large bowl, coat the cucumber slices with the rice wine vinegar, salt, and sugar.
3. Place a dish on top of the bowl to weight it down completely.
4. In another bowl, mix the eggplants, mirin rice wine, and miso paste. Let marinate for half an hour.

5. Close and flip the SmartSwitch to AIRFRY/STOVETOP. Select AIRFRY, set temperature to 390°F, and set time to 15 minutes (unit will need to preheat for 5 minutes, so set an external timer if desired). Press START/STOP to begin cooking.

6. When the unit is preheated and the time reaches 10 minutes, place the eggplants on the tray. Close the lid to begin cooking.

7. After 5 minutes, open the lid and toss the eggplants with silicone tipped tongs to ensure even cooking. Close the lid to continue cooking.

8. Fill the bottom of a serving bowl with rice and top with the eggplants and pickled cucumbers.

9. Place the spring onions and sesame seeds for garnish. Serve hot.

Nutrition: Calories: 230kcal; Fat: 3g; Carb: 0.1g; Protein: 9g

95.   Cauliflower, Chickpea, and Avocado Mash

Preparation Time: 10 minutes

Cooking Time: 5 minutes

Servings: 4

Ingredients:

- 1 medium head cauliflower, cut into florets
- 1 can chickpeas, drained and rinsed
- 1 tbsp. extravirgin olive oil
- 2 tbsps. lemon juice
- Salt and ground black pepper, to taste
- 4 flatbreads, toasted
- 2 ripe avocados, mashed

Directions:

1. Push in the legs on the Crisper Tray, then place the tray in the bottom of the pot. Spray the tray with cooking spray.

2. In a bowl, combine the chickpeas, cauliflower, lemon juice and olive oil. Season with salt and pepper as desired.

3. Close and flip the SmartSwitch to AIRFRY/STOVETOP. Select AIRFRY, set temperature to 390°F, and set time to 20 minutes (unit will need to preheat for 5 minutes, so set an external timer if desired). Press START/STOP to begin cooking.

4. When the unit is preheated and the time reaches 15 minutes, place the mixture on the tray. Close the lid to begin cooking.

5. Spread top of the flatbread along with the mashed avocado. Season with more pepper and salt and serve.

Nutrition: Calories: 212kcal; Fat: 1.45g; Carb: 2.56g; Protein: 7g

96.   Green Beans with Shallot

Preparation Time: 10 minutes

Cooking Time: 10 minutes

Servings: 4

Ingredients:

- ½ cup water, for steaming
- 2 tbsps. olive oil
- 1½ pounds (680 g) French green beans, stems removed and blanched
- ½ pound (227 g) shallots, peeled and cut into quarters
- 1 tbsp. salt
- ½ tsp. ground white pepper

Directions:

1. Pour ½ cup water into the pot. Push in the legs on the Crisper Tray, then place the tray in the bottom position in the pot.
2. Coat the vegetables evenly with the rest of the ingredients in a bowl. Then transfer the vegetables to the tray.
3. Close and flip the SmartSwitch to Rapid Cooker. Select STEAM & CRISP, set temperature to 375°F, and set time to 10 minutes. Press START/STOP to start cooking (the unit will steam for approx. 4 minutes before crisping).
4. With 5 minutes remaining, open the lid and toss the vegetables with tongs. Close the lid to continue cooking.
5. When cooking is complete, use tongs to remove the vegetables from the tray and serve hot.

Nutrition: Calories: 230kcal; Fat: 2.43g; Carb: 0.56g; Protein: 9g

97.   Mediterranean Air Fried Veggies

Preparation Time: 10 minutes

Cooking Time: 5 minutes

Servings: 4

Ingredients:

- cooking spray
- 1 large zucchini, sliced
- 1 cup cherry tomatoes, halved
- 1 parsnip, sliced
- 1 green pepper, sliced
- 1 carrot, sliced
- 1 tsp. mixed herbs
- 1 tsp. mustard

- 1 tsp. garlic purée
- 6 tbsps. olive oil
- Salt and ground black pepper, to taste

Directions:

1. Push in the legs on the Crisper Tray, then place the tray in the bottom of the pot. Spray the tray with cooking spray.

2. Mix all the ingredients in a bowl, making sure to coat the vegetables well.

3. Close and flip the SmartSwitch to AIRFRY/STOVETOP. Select AIRFRY, set temperature to 390°F, and set time to 15 minutes (unit will need to preheat for 5 minutes, so set an external timer if desired). Press START/STOP to begin cooking.

4. When the unit is preheated and the time reaches 10 minutes, place the vegetables on the tray. Close the lid to begin cooking.

5. After 5 minutes, open the lid and toss the vegetables with silicone tipped tongs to ensure even cooking. Close the lid to continue cooking.

6. When cooking is complete, serve hot.

Nutrition: Calories: 189kcal; Fat: 3g; Carb: 2g; Protein: 9g

98.   Potatoes with Zucchinis

Preparation Time: 10 minutes

Cooking Time: 15 minutes

Servings: 8

Ingredients:

- 2 potatoes, peeled and cubed
- 4 carrots, cut into chunks
- 1 head broccoli, cut into florets
- 4 zucchinis, sliced thickly
- Salt and ground black pepper, to taste
- ¼ cup olive oil
- 1 tbsp. dry onion powder

Directions:

1. Push in the legs on the Crisper Tray, then place the tray in the bottom of the pot. Spray the tray with cooking spray.

2. In a large basin, add all the ingredients and combine well.

3. Close and flip the SmartSwitch to AIRFRY/STOVETOP. Select AIRFRY, set temperature to 390°F, and set time to 30 minutes (unit will need to preheat for 5 minutes, so set an external timer if desired). Press START/STOP to begin cooking.

4. When the unit is preheated and the time reaches 25 minutes, place the vegetables on the tray. Close the lid to begin cooking.

5. After 10 minutes, open the lid and toss the vegetables with silicone tipped tongs to ensure even cooking. Close the lid to continue cooking. Serve warm.

Nutrition: Calories: 156kcal; Fat: 1.67g; Carb: 2g; Protein: 9g

99.   Gold Ravioli

Preparation Time: 10 minutes

Cooking Time: 6 minutes

Servings: 4

Ingredients:

- Cooking spray
- 8 ounces (227 g) ravioli
- ½ cup panko bread crumbs
- 2 tsps. nutritional yeast
- 1 tsp. dried basil
- 1 tsp. dried oregano
- 1 tsp. garlic powder

- Salt and ground black pepper, to taste
- ¼ cup aquafaba

Directions:

1. Push in the legs on the Crisper Tray, then place the tray in the bottom of the pot. Spray the tray with cooking spray and cover with aluminum foil.
2. Mix the panko bread crumbs, nutritional yeast, basil, oregano, and garlic powder. Combine with salt and pepper to taste.
3. Place the aquafaba in a separate bowl. Dunk the ravioli in the aquafaba before coating it in the panko mixture. Spritz with cooking spray.
4. Close and flip the SmartSwitch to AIRFRY/STOVETOP. Select AIRFRY, set temperature to 400°F, and set time to 11 minutes (unit will need to preheat for 5 minutes, so set an external timer if desired). Press START/STOP to begin cooking.
5. When the unit is preheated and the time reaches 6 minutes, place the ravioli on the tray. Close the lid to begin cooking.
6. After 3 minutes, open the lid and toss the ravioli with silicone tipped tongs to ensure even cooking. Close the lid to continue cooking.
7. When cooking is complete, serve hot.

Nutrition: Calories: 220kcal; Fat: 3g; Carb: 2g; Protein: 9g

100.   Blistered Shishito Peppers

Preparation Time: 10 minutes

Cooking Time: 8 minutes

Servings: 4

Ingredients:

Dipping Sauce:

- 1 cup sour cream
- 1 green onion (white and green parts), finely chopped
- 1 clove garlic, minced
- 2 tbsps. fresh lemon juice

Peppers:

- 8 ounces (227 g) shishito peppers
- 1 tbsp. vegetable oil
- 1 tsp. toasted sesame oil
- ½ tsp. toasted sesame seeds
- ¼ to ½ tsp. red pepper flakes
- Kosher salt and black pepper, to taste

Directions:

1. Push in the legs on the Crisper Tray, then place the tray in the bottom of the pot. Spray the tray with cooking spray.
2. In a small bowl, mix all the ingredients for the dipping sauce to combine well. Cover and refrigerate until serving time.
3. In a medium bowl, stir the peppers with the vegetable oil.
4. Close the lid and flip the SmartSwitch to AIRFRY/STOVETOP. Select AIRFRY, set temperature to 350°F, and set time to 13 minutes (unit will need to preheat for 5 minutes, so set an external timer if desired). Press START/STOP to begin cooking.
5. When the unit is preheated and the time reaches 8 minutes, place the peppers on the tray. Close the lid to begin cooking.
6. After 4 minutes, open the lid and toss the peppers with silicone tipped tongs to ensure even cooking. Close the lid to continue cooking.
7. When cooking is complete, transfer the peppers to a serving bowl. Pour the sesame oil and toss to coat well. Sprinkle with salt and pepper. Place the red pepper and sesame seeds and toss again.
8. Serve hot with the dipping sauce.

Nutrition: Calories: 198kcal; Fat: 2g; Carb: 3g; Protein: 5g

101. Creamy and Cheesy Spinach

Preparation Time: 15 minutes

Cooking Time: 19 minutes

Servings: 4

Ingredients:

- ½ cup water, for steaming
- Vegetable oil spray
- 1 (10ounce / 283g) package frozen spinach, thawed and squeezed dry
- ½ cup chopped onion
- ½ cup grated Parmesan cheese
- 4 ounces (113 g) cream cheese, diced
- 2 cloves garlic, minced
- ½ tsp. ground nutmeg
- 1 tsp. kosher salt
- 1 tsp. black pepper

Directions:

1. Pour ½ cup water into the pot. Push in the legs on the Crisper Tray, then place the tray in the bottom position in the pot. Spray a 8inch round baking pan with cooking spray.
2. In a medium bowl, combine the spinach, onion, garlic, cream cheese, nutmeg, salt, and pepper. Place the prepared pan and transfer on the tray.

3. Close the lid and flip the SmartSwitch to Rapid Cooker. Select STEAM & CRISP, set temperature to 350°F, and set time to 10 minutes. Press START/STOP to begin cooking (the unit will steam for approx. 4 minutes before crisping).

4. With 5 minutes remaining, open the lid and toss the spinach with tongs. Close the lid to continue cooking.

5. Open and stir to thoroughly Mix the cream cheese and spinach.

6. Place the Parmesan cheese on top. Bake for 5 minutes, or until the cheese has melted and browned.

7. Serve warm.

Nutrition: Calories: 230kcal; Fat: 3g; Carb: 2g; Protein: 9g

102.   Herbed Radishes

Preparation Time: 5 minutes

Cooking Time: 10 minutes

Servings: 2

Ingredients:

- cooking spray
- 1 pound (454 g) radishes
- 2 tbsps. unsalted butter, melted
- ½ tsp. dried parsley
- ½ tsp. garlic powder
- ¼ tsp. dried oregano

Directions:

7. Push in the legs on the Crisper Tray, then place the tray in the bottom of the pot. Spray the tray with cooking spray.

8. Prepare the radishes by cutting off their tops and bottoms and quartering them.

9. In a bowl, mix the butter, dried oregano, dried parsley, and garlic powder. Toss with the radishes to coat well.

10. Close the lid and flip the SmartSwitch to AIRFRY/STOVETOP. Select AIRFRY, set temperature to 390°F, and set time to 15 minutes (unit will need to preheat for 5 minutes, so set an external timer if desired). Press START/STOP to begin cooking.

11. When the unit is preheated and the time reaches 10 minutes, place the radishes on the tray. Close the lid to begin cooking.

12. After 5 minutes, open the lid and toss the radishes with silicone tipped tongs to ensure even cooking. Close the lid to continue cooking.

13. The radishes are ready when they turn brown.

14. Serve hot.

Nutrition: Calories: 123kcal; Fat: 3g; Carb: 2g; Protein: 8g

CHAPTER 7: Desserts

103.   Strawberry Cheesecake Bars

Preparation Time: 5 minutes

Cooking Time: 25 minutes

Servings: 16

Ingredients:

- 2 cups graham crackers
- 1/2 cup butter, melted
- 2 (8 ounce) packages cream cheese, softened
- 2/3 cup white sugar
- 2 eggs
- 2 tablespoons all-purpose flour
- 2 teaspoons vanilla extract
- 2 cups fresh strawberries, diced
- 1/4 cup strawberry preserves

Directions:

1. Preheat the Ninja Speedi Rapid Cooker to 375 degrees F (190 degrees C).
2. Place the graham crackers in a food processor and pulse until they are finely ground. Transfer the graham cracker crumbs to a medium bowl and stir in the melted butter until the mixture is evenly moistened. Press the mixture into the bottom of a greased 9x13inch baking pan.
3. In a separate bowl, beat together the cream cheese and sugar until light and fluffy. Crack the eggs and beat one at a time, then stir in the flour and vanilla extract. Spread the cream cheese mixture over the graham cracker crust.
4. Place the diced strawberries on top of the cream cheese layer and spoon the strawberry preserves over the top.
5. Bake in the preheated Ninja Speedi Rapid Cooker for 25 minutes, or until the top is lightly browned and the center is set.

Nutrition: Calories: 204kcal; Fat: 12g; Carb: 20g; Protein: 2g

104.   Chocolate Fondue

Preparation Time: 5 minutes

Cooking Time: 10 minutes

Servings: 8

Ingredients:

- 2 cups semisweet chocolate chips
- 1/2 cup heavy cream
- 2 tablespoons butter
- 1 tablespoon light corn syrup
- 1 teaspoon vanilla extract

Directions:

1. Place the chocolate chips, cream, butter and corn syrup in the Ninja Speedi Rapid Cooker. Lower heat and cook for 10 minutes, stirring once in a while.

2. Turn off heat and stir in the vanilla extract. Serve with fresh fruit or other dippers.

Nutrition: Calories: 226kcal; Fat: 15g; Carb: 20g; Protein: 3.2g

105.   Apple Cobbler

Preparation Time: 5 minutes

Cooking Time: 60 minutes

Servings: 8

Ingredients:

- 2 tablespoons butter
- 4 large apples, peeled, cored, and sliced
- 1/2 cup white sugar
- 1 teaspoon ground cinnamon
- 1/2 cup all-purpose flour
- 1/2 cup packed brown sugar
- 1/2 cup rolled oats
- 1/4 teaspoon salt
- 1/4 teaspoon ground nutmeg
- 1/4 cup butter, melted

Directions:

1. Grease the Ninja Speedi Rapid Cooker with the 2 tablespoons butter. Place the sliced apples in the cooker and sprinkle the white sugar and cinnamon over the top.

2. In a medium basin, mix together the flour, brown sugar, oats, salt, and nutmeg. Cut in the 1/4 cup melted butter until the mixture is crumbly. Spread the mixture over the top of the apples.

3. Conceal and cook on high for 2 hours, or until the apples are tender.

Nutrition: Calories: 222kcal; Fat: 7g; Carb: 38g; Protein: 2.4g

106.   Apple Crisp

Preparation Time: 5 minutes

Cooking Time: 60 minutes

Servings: 8

Ingredients:

- 4 large apples, peeled, cored, and sliced
- 1/4 cup white sugar
- 1 tablespoon ground cinnamon
- 1/2 cup all-purpose flour
- 1/2 cup packed brown sugar
- 1/2 cup rolled oats
- 1/4 teaspoon salt
- 1/4 teaspoon ground nutmeg
- 1/4 cup butter, melted

Directions:

1. Place the sliced apples in the Ninja Speedi Rapid Cooker and sprinkle the white sugar and cinnamon over the top.
2. In a medium basin, mix together the flour, brown sugar, oats, salt, and nutmeg. Cut in the 1/4 cup melted butter until the mixture is crumbly. Spread the mixture over the top of the apples.
3. Conceal and cook on high for 2 hours, or until the apples are tender.

Nutrition: Calories: 182kcal; Fat: 5.3g; Carb: 34g; Protein: 7g

107.   Rice Pudding

Preparation Time: 5 minutes

Cooking Time: 2 hours

Servings: 4

Ingredients:

- 1 cup white rice
- 2 cups milk
- 2 tablespoons butter
- 1/3 cup white sugar
- 1/4 teaspoon ground cinnamon
- 1/4 cup raisins
- 1/4 teaspoon vanilla extract

Directions:

1. Place the rice, milk, butter, sugar, and cinnamon in the Ninja Speedi Rapid Cooker. Conceal and cook on low for 2 to 3 hours, or until the rice is tender.
2. Once the rice is cooked, stir in the raisins and vanilla extract. Serve warm or chilled.

Nutrition: Calories: 207kcal; Fat: 7.1g; Carb: 32g; Protein: 4.3g

108. Banana Bread Pudding

Preparation Time: 5 minutes

Cooking Time: 1 hour

Servings: 8

Ingredients:

- 4 cups cubed day old bread
- 2 cups milk
- 1/2 cup white sugar
- 2 eggs, lightly beaten
- 2 ripe bananas, mashed
- 1 teaspoon vanilla extract
- 1/4 teaspoon ground cinnamon
- 1/4 teaspoon ground nutmeg
- 1/4 cup raisins

Directions:

1. Grease the Ninja Speedi Rapid Cooker with butter or nonstick cooking spray. Place the cubed bread in the cooker.
2. In a medium bowl, whisk together the milk, sugar, eggs, mashed bananas, vanilla extract, cinnamon, and nutmeg. Pour the mixture over the bread in the cooker. Stir in the raisins.
3. Conceal and cook on high for 1 1/2 hours, or until the pudding is set. Serve warm or chilled.

Nutrition: Calories: 195kcal; Fat: 3.7g; Carb: 34g; Protein: 5g

109. Chocolate Chip Bread Pudding

Preparation Time: 5 minutes

Cooking Time: 1 hour

Servings: 4

Ingredients:

- 4 cups cubed day old bread
- 2 cups milk
- 1/2 cup white sugar
- 2 eggs, lightly beaten
- 1/2 cup semisweet chocolate chips
- 1 teaspoon vanilla extract
- 1/4 teaspoon ground cinnamon
- 1/4 teaspoon ground nutmeg

Directions:

1. Grease the Ninja Speedi Rapid Cooker with butter or nonstick cooking spray. Place the cubed bread in the cooker.
2. In a medium bowl, whisk together the milk, sugar, eggs, chocolate chips, vanilla extract, cinnamon, and nutmeg. Pour the mixture over the bread in the cooker.
3. Cover and cook on high for 1 1/2 hours, or until the pudding is set. Serve warm or chilled.

Nutrition: Calories: 213kcal; Fat: 7g; Carb: 33g; Protein: 5.2g

110.   Vanilla Custard

Preparation Time: 5 minutes

Cooking Time: 1 hour

Servings: 6

Ingredients:

- 2 cups halfandhalf
- 1/2 cup white sugar
- 4 egg yolks
- 1 teaspoon vanilla extract
- 1/8 teaspoon salt

Directions:

1. Place the halfandhalf, sugar, egg yolks, vanilla extract, and salt in the Ninja Speedi Rapid Cooker. Stir until the sugar is dissolved.
2. Cover and cook on low for 1 1/2 to 2 hours, or until the custard is thickened. Serve warm or chilled.

Nutrition: Calories: 177kcal; Fat: 10.8g; Carb: 16g; Protein: 3.7g

111.   Apple Crumble Cake

Preparation Time: 5 minutes

Cooking Time: 25 minutes

Servings: 4

Ingredients:

- 2 cups all-purpose flour
- 1 cup white sugar
- 1 teaspoon baking powder
- ½ teaspoon baking soda
- ½ teaspoon salt
- ½ cup butter, melted
- 1 teaspoon vanilla extract
- 2 eggs
- 2 cups peeled and finely chopped apples

- 1 teaspoon ground cinnamon
- ½ cup chopped walnuts

Directions:

1. Preheat the Ninja Speedi Rapid Cooker to 350 degrees F (175 degrees C). Grease the inner pot.
2. In a large bowl, sift together the flour, sugar, baking powder, baking soda, and salt.
3. In a separate bowl, mix together the melted butter, vanilla, and eggs.
4. Pour the wet ingredients into the dry ingredients and mix until just combined.
5. Stir in the apples, cinnamon, and walnuts.
6. Pour the batter into the prepared inner pot.
7. Cover and cook on high pressure for 25 minutes.
8. Allow the pressure to release naturally.
9. Serve warm with ice cream or whipped cream.

Nutrition: Calories: 230kcal; Fat: 10g; Carb: 30g; Protein: 4g

112. Gingerbread Pudding Cake

Preparation Time: 5 minutes

Cooking Time: 25 minutes

Servings: 4

Ingredients:

- 2 cups all-purpose flour
- 2 teaspoons ground ginger
- 1 teaspoon ground cinnamon
- ½ teaspoon ground nutmeg
- ½ teaspoon baking powder
- ½ teaspoon baking soda
- ¼ teaspoon salt
- 1 cup light brown sugar
- ½ cup butter, melted
- 1 cup molasses
- 2 eggs
- ½ cup water

Directions:

1. Preheat the Ninja Speedi Rapid Cooker to 350 degrees F (175 degrees C). Grease the inner pot.
2. In a large bowl, sift together the flour, ginger, cinnamon, nutmeg, baking powder, baking soda, and salt.
3. In a separate bowl, mix together the melted butter, brown sugar, molasses, eggs, and water.
4. Pour the wet ingredients into the dry ingredients and mix until just combined.

5. Pour the batter into the prepared inner pot.

6. Cover and cook on high pressure for 25 minutes.

7. Allow the pressure to release naturally.

8. Serve warm with ice cream or whipped cream.

Nutrition: Calories: 315kcal; Fat: 8g; Carb: 52g; Protein: 4g

113.　　Chocolate Fudge Cake

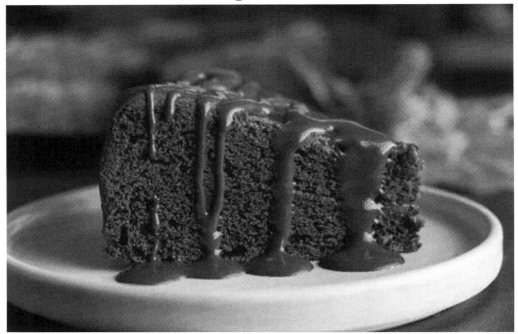

Preparation Time: 5 minutes

Cooking Time: 25 minutes

Servings: 4

Ingredients:

- 2 cups all-purpose flour
- 2/3 cup cocoa powder
- 1 teaspoon baking powder
- ½ teaspoon baking soda
- ½ teaspoon salt
- 1 cup light brown sugar
- ½ cup butter, melted
- 1 teaspoon vanilla extract
- 2 eggs
- 1 cup milk
- 12 ounces semisweet chocolate chips

Directions:

1. Preheat the Ninja Speedi Rapid Cooker to 350 degrees F (175 degrees C). Grease the inner pot.
2. In a large bowl, sift together the flour, cocoa powder, baking powder, baking soda, and salt.
3. In a separate bowl, mix together the melted butter, brown sugar, vanilla, eggs, and milk.
4. Pour wet ingredients into the dry ingredients and mix until just combined.
5. Stir in the chocolate chips.
6. Pour the batter into the prepared inner pot.
7. Cover and cook on high pressure for 25 minutes.
8. Allow the pressure to release naturally.
9. Serve warm with whipped cream or ice cream.

Nutrition: Calories: 516kcal; Fat: 25g; Carb: 63g; Protein: 8g

114.   Cinnamon Swirl Cake

Preparation Time: 5 minutes

Cooking Time: 25 minutes

Servings: 4

Ingredients:

- 2 cups all-purpose flour
- 1 cup white sugar
- 1 teaspoon baking powder
- ½ teaspoon baking soda
- ½ teaspoon salt
- ½ cup butter, melted
- 1 teaspoon vanilla extract
- 2 eggs
- 1 cup milk
- 2 tablespoons ground cinnamon

Directions:

1. Preheat the Ninja Speedi Rapid Cooker to 350 degrees F (175 degrees C). Grease the inner pot.
2. In a large basin, sift together the flour, sugar, baking powder, baking soda, and salt.
3. In a separate bowl, mix together the melted butter, vanilla, eggs, and milk.
4. Pour wet ingredients into the dry ingredients and mix until just combined.
5. Pour 1/2 of the batter into the prepared inner pot.
6. Sprinkle the cinnamon over the batter.
7. Pour the remaining batter over the cinnamon and swirl with a knife.
8. Cover and cook on high pressure for 25 minutes.
9. Allow the pressure to release naturally.

10. Serve warm with whipped cream or ice cream.

Nutrition: Calories: 250kcal; Fat: 10g; Carb: 35g; Protein: 4g

115.   Blueberry Cobbler

Preparation Time: 5 minutes

Cooking Time: 25 minutes

Servings: 4

Ingredients:

- 2 cups all-purpose flour
- 1 cup white sugar
- 1 teaspoon baking powder
- ½ teaspoon baking soda
- ½ teaspoon salt
- ½ cup butter, melted
- 1 teaspoon vanilla extract
- 2 eggs
- 2 cups fresh or frozen blueberries
- 1 teaspoon ground cinnamon
- 2 tablespoons white sugar

Directions:

1. Preheat the Ninja Speedi Rapid Cooker to 350 degrees F (175 degrees C). Grease the inner pot.
2. In a large basin, sift together the flour, sugar, baking powder, baking soda, and salt.
3. In a separate bowl, mix together the melted butter, vanilla, and eggs.
4. Pour wet ingredients into the dry ingredients and mix until just combined.
5. Stir in the blueberries.
6. Pour the batter into the prepared inner pot.
7. In a small basin, mix together the cinnamon and sugar.
8. Sprinkle the cinnamon sugar mixture over the batter.
9. Cover and cook on high pressure for 25 minutes.
10. Allow the pressure to release naturally.
11. Serve warm with ice cream or whipped cream.

Nutrition: Calories: 250kcal; Fat: 10g; Carb: 35g; Protein: 4g

116.   Banana Bread

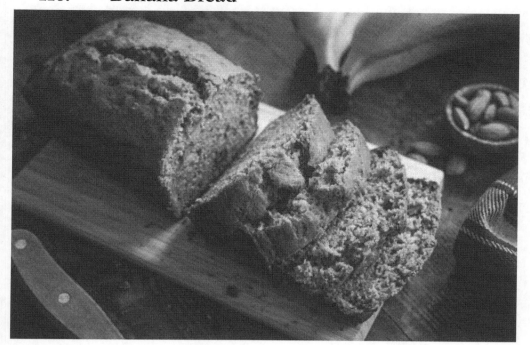

Preparation Time: 5 minutes

Cooking Time: 25 minutes

Servings: 4

Ingredients:

- 2 cups all-purpose flour
- 1 teaspoon baking powder
- ½ teaspoon baking soda
- ½ teaspoon salt
- ½ cup butter, melted
- 1 teaspoon vanilla extract
- 2 eggs
- 2 cups mashed ripe bananas
- ½ cup chopped walnuts (optional)

Directions:

1.   Preheat the Ninja Speedi Rapid Cooker to 350 degrees F (175 degrees C). Grease the inner pot.
2.   In a large bowl, sift together the flour, baking powder, baking soda, and salt.
3.   In a separate bowl, mix together the melted butter, vanilla, eggs, and mashed bananas.
4.   Pour the wet ingredients into the dry ingredients and mix until just combined.
5.   Stir in the walnuts, if using.
6.   Pour the batter into the prepared inner pot.
7.   Cover and cook on high pressure for 25 minutes.

8. Allow the pressure to release naturally.

9. Serve warm with ice cream or whipped cream.

Nutrition: Calories: 250kcal; Fat: 10g; Carb: 35g; Protein: 4g

117.   Peach Cobbler

Preparation Time: 5 minutes

Cooking Time: 15 minutes

Servings: 4

Ingredients:

- 2 cups all-purpose flour
- 1 cup white sugar
- 1 teaspoon baking powder
- ½ teaspoon baking soda
- ½ teaspoon salt
- ½ cup butter, melted
- 1 teaspoon vanilla extract
- 2 eggs
- 2 cups peeled and chopped fresh peaches
- 2 tablespoons white sugar
- 1 teaspoon ground cinnamon

Directions:

1. Preheat the Ninja Speedi Rapid Cooker to 350 degrees F (175 degrees C). Grease the inner pot.

2. In a large bowl, sift together the flour, sugar, baking powder, baking soda, and salt.

3. In a separate bowl, mix together the melted butter, vanilla, and eggs.

4. Pour the wet ingredients into the dry ingredients and mix until just combined.

5. Stir in the peaches.

6. Pour the batter into the prepared inner pot.

7. In a small bowl, mix together the sugar and cinnamon.

8. Sprinkle the cinnamon sugar mixture over the batter.

9. Cover and cook on high pressure for 25 minutes.

10. Allow the pressure to release naturally.

11. Serve warm with ice cream or whipped cream.

Nutrition: Calories: 250kcal; Fat: 10g; Carb: 35g; Protein: 4g

118.   Cherry Cobbler

Preparation Time: 5 minutes

Cooking Time: 25 minutes

Servings: 4

Ingredients:

- 2 cups all-purpose flour
- 1 cup white sugar
- 1 teaspoon baking powder
- ½ teaspoon baking soda
- ½ teaspoon salt
- ½ cup butter, melted
- 1 teaspoon vanilla extract
- 2 eggs
- 2 cups pitted and chopped fresh or frozen cherries
- 2 tablespoons white sugar
- 1 teaspoon ground cinnamon

Directions:

1. Preheat the Ninja Speedi Rapid Cooker to 350 degrees F (175 degrees C). Grease the inner pot.
2. In a large bowl, sift together the flour, sugar, baking powder, baking soda, and salt.
3. In a separate bowl, mix together the melted butter, vanilla, and eggs.
4. Pour wet ingredients into the dry ingredients and mix until just combined.
5. Stir in the cherries.
6. Pour the batter into the prepared inner pot.
7. In a small bowl, mix together the sugar and cinnamon.
8. Sprinkle the cinnamon sugar mixture over the batter.
9. Cover and cook on high pressure for 25 minutes.
10. Allow the pressure to release naturally.
11. Serve warm with whipped cream or ice cream.

Nutrition: Calories: 250kcal; Fat: 10g; Carb: 36g; Protein: 9.4g

119.   Carrot Cake

Preparation Time: 5 minutes

Cooking Time: 15 minutes

Servings: 4

Ingredients:

- 2 cups all-purpose flour
- 1 cup white sugar
- 1 teaspoon baking powder
- ½ teaspoon baking soda
- ½ teaspoon salt

- ½ cup butter, melted
- 1 teaspoon vanilla extract
- 2 eggs
- 2 cups grated carrots
- ½ cup chopped walnuts
- 1 teaspoon ground cinnamon

Directions:

1. Preheat the Ninja Speedi Rapid Cooker to 350 degrees F (175 degrees C). Grease the inner pot.
2. In a large basin, sift together the flour, sugar, baking powder, baking soda, and salt.
3. In a separate bowl, mix together the melted butter, vanilla, and eggs.
4. Pour wet ingredients into the dry ingredients and mix until just combined.
5. Stir in the carrots, walnuts, and cinnamon.
6. Pour the batter into the prepared inner pot.
7. Cover and cook on high pressure for 25 minutes.
8. Allow the pressure to release naturally.
9. Serve warm with whipped cream or ice cream.

Nutrition: Calories: 260kcal; Fat: 13g; Carb: 36g; Protein: 9.4g

120. Strawberry Cake

Preparation Time: 5 minutes

Cooking Time: 15 minutes

Servings: 4

Ingredients:

- 2 cups all-purpose flour
- 1 cup white sugar
- 1 teaspoon baking powder
- ½ teaspoon baking soda
- ½ teaspoon salt
- ½ cup butter, melted
- 1 teaspoon vanilla extract
- 2 eggs
- 2 cups chopped fresh strawberries

Directions:

1. Preheat the Ninja Speedi Rapid Cooker to 350 degrees F (175 degrees C). Grease the inner pot.
2. In a large basin, sift together the flour, sugar, baking powder, baking soda, and salt.
3. In a separate bowl, mix together the melted butter, vanilla, and eggs.
4. Pour wet ingredients into the dry ingredients and mix until just combined.

5. Stir in the strawberries.
6. Pour the batter into the prepared inner pot.
7. Cover and cook on high pressure for 25 minutes.
8. Allow the pressure to release naturally.
9. Serve warm with whipped cream or ice cream.

Nutrition: Calories: 245kcal; Fat: 13g; Carb: 35g; Protein: 4g

Conclusion

This Cookbook has proven to be an invaluable resource for home cooks. With its simple yet comprehensive instructions, it provides a great foundation for creating delicious meals quickly and easily. The recipes are easy to follow, specially made for the inexperienced cook, and feature ingredients that are readily available and accessible. This cookbook also offers tips and tricks to help make cooking more efficient, as well as nutritional information about each recipe. In addition, it shows how to cook with the Ninja Speedi Rapid Cooker, which makes cooking faster and easier than ever before! Thanks to this incredible book, home cooks everywhere can enjoy delicious meals with minimal effort in little time.

In conclusion, the Ninja Speedi Rapid Cooker Cookbook is a great resource for anyone who wants to make quick and delicious meals. It provides an abundance of recipes, from breakfast to main dishes and even desserts, that can be made in minutes with the Ninja Speedi Rapid Cooker. The recipes are easy to follow and include nutritional information for each recipe. Additionally, the cookbook features helpful tips for using the cooker, as well as safety warnings. With this cookbook by your side, you will be able to create meals that are not only delicious but also healthy and nutritious. So pick up your copy of Ninja Speedi Rapid Cooker Cookbook today and get ready to enjoy fast, flavorful meals that you can feel good about eating on a daily basis!

Printed in Great Britain
by Amazon

33568045R00057